Advances in Microsurgical Reconstruction in the Upper Extremity

Editors

HARVEY CHIM
KEVIN C. CHUNG

HAND CLINICS

www.hand.theclinics.com

Consulting Editor
KEVIN C. CHUNG

May 2024 • Volume 40 • Number 2

ELSEVIER

1600 John F. Kennedy Boulevard • Suite 1800 • Philadelphia, Pennsylvania, 19103-2899

http://www.theclinics.com

HAND CLINICS Volume 40, Number 2
May 2024 ISSN 0749-0712, ISBN-13: 978-0-443-13013-7

Editor: Megan Ashdown
Developmental Editor: Akshay Samson

Hand Clinics (ISSN 0749-0712) is published quarterly by Elsevier Inc., 360 Park Avenue South, New York, NY 10010-1710. Months of publication are February, May, August, and November. Business and Editorial Offices: 1600 John F. Kennedy Blvd., Ste. 1800, Philadelphia, PA 19103-2899. Customer Service Office: 3251 Riverport Lane, Maryland Heights, MO 63043. Periodicals postage paid at New York, NY and at additional mailing offices. Subscription price is $457.00 per year (domestic individuals), $100.00 per year (domestic students/residents), $506.00 per year (Canadian individuals), $579.00 per year (international individuals), $256.00 (international students/residents), and $100.00 (Canadian students/residents). For institutional access pricing please contact Customer Service via the contact information below. Foreign air speed delivery is included in all *Clinics* subscription prices. All prices are subject to change without notice. **POSTMASTER:** Send address changes to *Hand Clinics*, Elsevier Health Sciences Division, Subscription Customer Service, 3251 Riverport Lane, Maryland Heights, MO 63043. Customer Service (orders, claims, online, change of address): Elsevier Health Sciences Division, Subscription **Customer Service, 3251 Riverport Lane, Maryland Heights, MO 63043. Tel: 1-800-654-2452 (U.S. and Canada); 314-447-8871 (outside U.S. and Canada). Fax: 314-447-8029. E-mail: journalscustomerservice-usa@elsevier.com (for print support); journalsonlinesupport-usa@elsevier.com (for online support).**

Reprints. For copies of 100 or more of articles in this publication, please contact the Commercial Reprints Department, Elsevier Inc., 360 Park Avenue South, New York, New York 10010-1710. Tel.: 212-633-3874; Fax: 212-633-3820; E-mail: reprints@elsevier.com.

Hand Clinics is covered in *MEDLINE/PubMed (Index Medicus)*, *Current Contents/Clinical Medicine*, *EMBASE/Excerpta Medica*, and *ISI/BIOMED*.

Contributors

CONSULTING EDITOR

KEVIN C. CHUNG, MD, MS
William C. Grabb Distinguished University Professor of Surgery, Charles B.G. de Nancrede Professor of Surgery, Professor of Plastic Surgery and Orthopaedic Surgery, Chief of Hand Surgery, Department of Surgery, Section of Plastic Surgery, Michigan Medicine, Assistant Dean for Faculty Affairs, Associate Director of Global REACH, University of Michigan Medical School, Director, University of Michigan Comprehensive Hand Center, University of Michigan, University of Michigan Health System, Ann Arbor, Michigan, USA

EDITORS

HARVEY CHIM, MD
Professor, Division of Plastic Surgery and Neurosurgery, Department of Surgery, University of Florida College of Medicine, Gainesville, Florida, USA

KEVIN C. CHUNG, MD, MS
William C. Grabb Distinguished University Professor of Surgery, Charles B.G. de Nancrede Professor of Surgery, Professor of Plastic Surgery and Orthopaedic Surgery, Chief of Hand Surgery, Department of Surgery, Section of Plastic Surgery, Michigan Medicine, Assistant Dean for Faculty Affairs, Associate Director of Global REACH, University of Michigan Medical School, Director, University of Michigan Comprehensive Hand Center, University of Michigan, University of Michigan Health System, Ann Arbor, Michigan, USA

AUTHORS

WIDYA ADIDHARMA, MD
Resident Physician, Section of Plastic Surgery, Department of Surgery, University of Michigan Medical School, Ann Arbor, Michigan, USA

JENNIFER BAI, MD
Integrated Plastic Surgery Resident, Division of Plastic and Reconstructive Surgery, Department of Surgery, Northwestern University Feinberg School of Medicine, Northwestern University, Chicago, Illinois, USA

CHIHENA HANSINI BANDA, MD, PhD
Head, Plastic and Reconstructive Surgery Unit, Department of Surgery, University Teaching Hospital, Lusaka, Zambia

CALEB W. BARNHILL, MD
Plastic Surgery Resident, Division of Plastic and Reconstructive Surgery, University of Colorado Hospital Anschutz Medical Center, Aurora, Colorado, USA

YANIS BERKANE, MD, MSc
Fellow, Department of Plastic, Reconstructive and Aesthetic Surgery, CHU Rennes, Rennes University, Rennes, France; Vascularized Composite Allotransplantation Laboratory, Massachusetts General Hospital, Harvard Medical School, Boston, Massachusetts, USA; UMR U1236-MICMAC, Immunology and Cell Therapy Lab, Rennes University Hospital, Rennes, France

JORGE G. BORETTO, MD
Head, Hand and Upper Extremity Surgery Department, Prof. Dr. "Carlos Ottolenghi Institute", Hospital Italiano de Buenos Aires, Buenos Aires, Argentina

XAVIER CHALHOUB, MBBS, BSc, MRCS
Specialty Registrar, Department of Plastic and Reconstructive Surgery, Royal Free Hospital, Royal Free London NHS Foundation Trust, London, United Kingdom

HARVEY CHIM, MD
Professor, Division of Plastic Surgery and
Neurosurgery, Department of Surgery,
University of Florida College of Medicine,
Gainesville, Florida, USA

JOHNNY CHUIENG-YI LU, MD, MSCI
Associate Professor, Department of Plastic
and Reconstructive Surgery, Chang Gung
Memorial Hospital, Taipei – Linkou, Taoyuan
City, Taiwan

KEVIN C. CHUNG, MD, MS
William C. Grabb Distinguished University
Professor of Surgery, Charles B.G. de
Nancrede Professor of Surgery, Professor of
Plastic Surgery and Orthopaedic Surgery,
Chief of Hand Surgery, Department of Surgery,
Section of Plastic Surgery, Michigan Medicine,
Assistant Dean for Faculty Affairs, Associate
Director of Global REACH, University of
Michigan Medical School, Director, University
of Michigan Comprehensive Hand Center,
University of Michigan, University of Michigan
Health System, Ann Arbor, Michigan, USA

DAVID CHWEI-CHIN CHUANG, MD
Professor, Department of Plastic and
Reconstructive Surgery, Chang Gung
Memorial Hospital, Taipei – Linkou, Taoyuan
City, Taiwan

CRISTIN L. COQUILLARD, MD
Surgeon, Integrated Plastic Surgery Resident,
Division of Plastic and Reconstructive Surgery,
Department of Surgery, Northwestern
University Feinberg School of Medicine,
Northwestern University, Chicago, Illinois, USA

SOUMEN DAS DE, MBBS, FRCS, MPH
Consultant, Department of Hand and
Reconstructive Microsurgery, National
University Health System, Singapore

MARCELO ROSA DE REZENDE, MD, PhD
Chief, Hand Surgery and Reconstructive
Microsurgery Group of the Institute of
Orthopedics and Traumatology, Clinics
Hospital of University of Sao Paulo, São Paulo,
Brazil

RUBEN DUKAN, MD, MSc
Department of Hand, Upper Limb and
Peripheral Nerve Surgery, Georges-Pompidou

European Hospital (HEGP), Department of
Orthopaedics, Georges Pompidou European
Hospital, Paris, France

**DOMINIC FURNISS, DM, MA, MBBCh,
FRCS(Plast)**
Professor, Botnar Research Centre and
Honorary Consultant, Professor, Department
of Plastic and Reconstructive Surgery, Nuffield
Orthopaedic Centre, Oxford University
Hospitals NHS Foundation Trust, Oxford,
United Kingdom

RICCARDO GIORGINO, MD
Fellow, Residency Program in Orthopaedics
and Traumatology, University of Milan, IRCCS
Istituto Ortopedico Galeazzi, Milan, Italy;
Plastic Surgery Research Laboratory, Wellman
Center for Photomedicine, Massachusetts
General Hospital, Harvard Medical School,
Boston, Massachusetts, USA

MARK A. GREYSON, MD
Assistant Professor, Section of Hand and Wrist
Surgery, Co-Director Extremity Microsurgery,
University of Colorado Hospital and Anschutz
Medical Center, Aurora, Colorado, USA

KOTA HAYASHI, MD
Department of Plastic and Reconstructive
Surgery, Chang Gung Memorial Hospital,
Taipei – Linkou, Taoyuan City, Taiwan

FERNANDO HOLC, MD
Hand and Upper Extremity Surgery
Department, Prof. Dr. "Carlos Ottolenghi
Institute", Hospital Italiano de Buenos Aires,
Buenos Aires, Argentina

YUN-HUAN HSIEH, MBBS, MS(PRS)
Department of Plastic and Reconstructive
Surgery, Chang Gung Memorial Hospital,
Chang Gung Medical College and Chang Gung
University, Taoyuan, Taiwan; Department of
Plastic and Reconstructive Surgery, St. Vincent
Private Hospital, East Melbourne, Australia

CHUNG-CHEN HSU, MD
Associate Professor, Department of Plastic
and Reconstructive Surgery, Chang Gung
Memorial Hospital, Chang Gung Medical
College and Chang Gung University, Taoyuan,
Taiwan

RAQUEL BERNARDELLI IAMAGUCHI, MD, MSc, PhD
Hand Surgery and Reconstructive Microsurgery Group of the Institute of Orthopedics and Traumatology, Clinics Hospital of University of Sao Paulo, São Paulo, Brazil

MATTHEW L. IORIO, MD
Professor, Division of Plastic and Reconstructive Surgery, Professor, Director, Plastic and Reconstructive Surgery Hand Surgery Service, Chief, Orthoplastics, Wound, and Nerve Surgery, Co-Director, Extremity Microsurgery, Co-Director, Wound Care Program, University of Colorado Hospital and Anschutz Medical Center, Aurora, Colorado, USA

RYOHEI ISHIURA, MD, PhD
Assistant Professor, Department of Plastic and Reconstructive Surgery, Graduate School of Medicine, Mie University, Tsu, Japan

SAW SIAN KHOO, MBChB
Consultant Orthopaedic Surgeon, National Orthopaedic Centre of Excellence for Research and Learning (NOCERAL), Department of Orthopaedic Surgery, Faculty of Medicine, Universiti Malaya, Kuala Lumpur, Malaysia

JASON H. KO, MD, MBA
Professor, Division of Plastic and Reconstructive Surgery, Departments of Surgery and Orthopaedic Surgery, Northwestern University Feinberg School of Medicine, Northwestern University, Chicago, Illinois, USA

ALEXANDRE G. LELLOUCH, MD, PhD
Lecturer, Vascularized Composite Allotransplantation Laboratory, Massachusetts General Hospital, Harvard Medical School, Boston, Massachusetts, USA

CHENG-HUNG LIN, MD, MBA, FACS
Professor, Department of Plastic and Reconstructive Surgery, Chang Gung Memorial Hospital, Chang Gung Medical College and Chang Gung University, Taoyuan, Taiwan

MARKOS MARDOURIAN, BS
Medical Student, Division of Plastic and Reconstructive Surgery, University of Florida College of Medicine, Gainesville, Florida, USA

TOMMY NAI-JEN CHANG, MD
Professor, Department of Plastic and Reconstructive Surgery, Chang Gung Memorial Hospital, Taipei – Linkou, Taoyuan City, Taiwan

MITSUNAGA NARUSHIMA, MD, PhD, FACS
Professor and Chief, Department of Plastic and Reconstructive Surgery, Graduate School of Medicine, Mie University, Tsu, Japan

ZHI YANG NG, MBChB, MRCS, PgDip, PhD
Specialty Registrar, Department of Plastic and Reconstructive Surgery, John Radcliffe Hospital, Oxford University Hospitals NHS Foundation Trust, Headington, Oxford, United Kingdom

KWANG HYUN PARK, MD
Senior Researcher, W Institute for Hand and Reconstructive Microsurgery, W General Hospital, Daegu, South Korea

RAMIN SHEKOUHI, MD
Research Fellow, Division of Plastic and Reconstructive Surgery, Department of Surgery, University of Florida College of Medicine, Gainesville, Florida, USA

MAKOTO SHIRAISHI, MD, PhD
Chief Resident, Department of Plastic and Reconstructive Surgery, Graduate School of Medicine, University of Tokyo, Tokyo, Japan

XIAO FANG SHEN, MD
Consultant Orthopaedic Surgeon, Department of Pediatric Orthopaedics, Children's Hospital of Soochow University, Suzhou, Jiangsu, China

ISAAC SMITH, BA
Medical Student, Division of Plastic and Reconstructive Surgery, University of Florida College of Medicine, Gainesville, Florida, USA

PEDRO BRONENBERG VICTORICA, MD
Associate Physician, Hand and Upper Extremity Surgery Department, Prof. Dr. "Carlos Ottolenghi Institute", Hospital Italiano de Buenos Aires, Buenos Aires, Argentina

HAO-I WEI, MD
Professor, Department of Plastic and Reconstructive Surgery, Chang Gung Memorial Hospital, Chang Gung Medical College and Chang Gung University, Taoyuan, Taiwan

SANG HYUN WOO, MD, PhD
President, W Institute for Hand and
Reconstructive Microsurgery, W General
Hospital, Daegu, South Korea

SOO JIN WOO, MD
W Institute for Hand and Reconstructive
Microsurgery, W General Hospital, Daegu,
South Korea

Contents

The upper extremity has unique functional and aesthetic requirements. Reconstruction of upper extremity soft tissue defects should ideally provide coverage for vital structures, facilitate early mobilization, be thin and pliable to match its slim contour, and reestablish sensation. Perforator flaps can be raised on the superficial fascia, which creates a thin and pliable yet durable and supple flap option to match the contour and functional needs of the upper extremity. Comparisons to traditional reconstructive methods should be performed to assess whether these innovations in microsurgical reconstruction of upper extremity defects provide an improved functional and aesthetic benefit over traditional methods.

Accurate preoperative localization of dominant perforators provides crucial information about their location and diameter, leading to reduced surgical time, improved flap viability, and decreased complications. Ultrasound has increased in popularity in recent years, with the advantages of providing reproducible, accurate, cost-effective, and real-time information while reducing radiation exposure. Precise preoperative mapping of perforators allows for rapid and safe elevation of suprafascial, thin, and superthin flaps. This review focuses on the role of ultrasound as a tool for preoperative flap planning in the upper extremities.

The superficial circumflex iliac artery perforator (SCIP) flap is thin, pliable tissue well suited for reconstruction of injuries of the hand and upper extremity. Based upon perforators from the superficial circumflex iliac artery, the SCIP flap has advantages over the traditional groin flap due to reduced need for secondary procedures and improved donor site morbidity This article offers a detailed exploration of the SCIP flap design and technique, its advantages over traditional methods, and its potential applications in reconstructive surgery. Post-operative care and critical points are also discussed, and case examples are provided to guide readers through the intricacies of the technique, emphasizing the surgical skill and precision required for successful implementation.

The profunda artery perforator (PAP) flap provides a good option for hand and upper extremity reconstruction. The reliable quality, caliber, and number of perforators in the posteromedial thigh support large flaps with long pedicles. The PAP flap has been widely used for breast reconstruction, although its use in the extremities has been slower to catch on due to the bulk and thickness of the subcutaneous tissue. The authors discuss evolution of thin flaps and our application of the thin and super-thin PAP flap for upper extremity reconstruction.

Upper extremity reconstruction remains challenging due to the high functional and esthetic demands of this location. The anterolateral thigh (ALT) flap is a workhorse flap for microsurgical reconstruction of the upper extremity and can be elevated in various planes depending on desired thickness of the flap. Microsurgical reconstruction of the upper extremity often benefits from a thin flap that can resurface the extremity, which can provide improved functional and esthetic outcomes. This article reviews the anatomy, preoperative planning, and operative technique, as well as presents 4 cases to illustrate the outcomes and benefits of thin and thinned ALT flaps.

The free medial sural artery perforator (MSAP) flap is a recently popularized flap. It has evolved from a composite myocutaneous flap to a pedicled perforator flap for lower limb reconstruction. It is also a versatile free perforator flap for extremity and head and neck reconstruction. The diversity of the flap designs with options for harvest of non-vascularized grafts enhances the versatility for hand and upper limb reconstruction. The adjunctive use of endoscopy and indocyanine green fluorescence imaging studies can assist and demystify the flap anatomy. The authors present their experience using free MSAP flaps for complex mutilated hand and upper extremity reconstruction.

Soft tissue defects of the hand may result from trauma, infection, vascular disease, and after resection of tumors. Microsurgery has evolved to a stage where it is relatively commonplace today but procedures such as free flaps still incur significant time, manpower, cost, and material resources. The aim of this article is to articulate the specific situations in hand reconstruction when microsurgery is superior to non-microsurgical reconstructive options. The benefits of microsurgical reconstruction include a variety of important metrics, such as improved function, better tissue match, less donor site morbidity, and reduced downtime for the patient.

Vascular malformations in the extremities are a common site of occurrence; arteriovenous malformations (AVMs) are the least frequent of all vascular malformations, estimated at 5% to 20%. The first step in management is to perform a thorough clinical examination. Symptoms are assessed, and staging is performed using the Schobinger classification. Next, ultrasonography and contrast-enhanced computed tomography are used to confirm the diagnosis of AVM and to confirm the extent of the malformation. Surgery is the first-line treatment and reconstruction is performed. In cases where surgery is not feasible, embolization and sclerotherapy may be used to alleviate symptoms.

 Video content accompanies this article at http://www.hand.theclinics.com

Microsurgery is undoubtedly the pinnacle of hand surgery. Significant advancement in recent years has stretched the indications for toe-to-hand transfer in both acquired and congenital hand defects to restore function, esthetics, and motion, with minimal morbidity to the donor site. There is no one fixed microsurgical transfer technique but a surgeon's versatility and innovation in using what one could spare because each case is unique. Esthetic refinements and reducing donor site morbidities have taken a front seat in recent years. We present a few cases to put forward the senior author's preferred techniques with this objective in mind.

The foot contains a unique collection of tissue types that can be used in the reconstruction of the hand. Numerous reconstructive options have been presented, some of which have been adopted, such as modifications to procedures that have been described in the past or even newly developed options for hand reconstruction. It is possible to reconstruct missing fingers and other hand structures using tissues taken from the foot rather than removing healthy tissue from a hand that has already been injured. This makes it possible to avoid having healthy tissue removed from an injured hand.

 Video content accompanies this article at http://www.hand.theclinics.com.

Traumatic brachial plexus injury is the most common indication for functional free muscle transfer, and elbow flexion recovery is the functional target, followed by shoulder stability and hand reanimation. In this article, we provide a literature review of functional free muscle transfer (FFMT) for adult traumatic brachial plexus injuries and the surgical technical recommendations to achieve the best functional results with FFMT for adult traumatic brachial plexus injuries.

 Video content accompanies this article at http://www.hand.theclinics.com.

Volkmann ischemic contracture (VIC) is a devastating condition that results from neglected compartment syndrome, which leads to prolonged ischemia, irreversible tissue necrosis, and various degrees of muscle and nerve damage, causing serious motor and sensory functional implications for the limb and a spectrum of diseases associated with worsening deformities. A thorough understanding of the anatomy and VIC pathophysiology is needed to plan an appropriate strategy. Functioning free muscle transplantation (FFMT) can restore finger movement in a paralyzed limb but requires a three-staged approach to maximize the benefits of FFMT, leading to meaningful finger extrinsic function.

The advent of supermicrosurgery has led to an increasing interest in the surgical management of lymphedema through the reconstruction of the lymphatic network, that is, the physiologic approach. Broadly, this can be divided into 2 main techniques: lymphaticovenous anastomosis and lymph node transfer. In the United Kingdom, the British Lymphology Society does not provide any recommendations on surgical management. Moreover, surgical treatment of lymphedema is not widely practiced within the National Health Service due to low-certainty evidence. Herein, we discuss our experience in physiologic reconstruction for lymphedema.

For major upper limb defects, a wide range of established pedicled and free flap options can be used. These include the latissimus dorsi/thoracodorsal artery perforator, lateral arm, posterior interosseous artery, rectus abdominis, gracilis, and anterolateral thigh flaps. Technical proficiency is essential, and favorable success rates in terms of functional and esthetic outcomes can be achieved. Herein, alternative flap options (both pedicled and free) are introduced and discussed through a few illustrative case examples.

In hand and upper extremity replantation surgery, simultaneous free flap reconstruction restores the physiologic circulation to the amputated part, ensuring its survival, and promotes wound healing through anatomic restoration. Especially in digit replantation, an arterialized venous flap serves to reconstruct both vessel and soft tissue defects simultaneously. Delayed free flap reconstruction aims to enhance both functional improvement and cosmetic acceptance in a successfully replanted part using flaps that include functioning muscle, bone, joint, nerve, and soft tissue.

HAND CLINICS

SERIES OF RELATED INTEREST:

Clinics in Plastic Surgery
www.plasticsurgery.theclinics.com

Orthopedic Clinics of North America
www.orthopedic.theclinics.com

Clinics in Sports Medicine
www.sportsmed.theclinics.com

THE CLINICS ARE AVAILABLE ONLINE!
Access your subscription at:
www.theclinics.com

Preface

Innovations in Microsurgical Reconstruction in the Upper Extremity

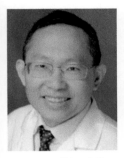 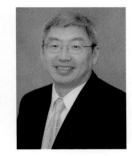

Harvey Chim, MD   Kevin C. Chung, MD, MS

Editors

Reconstruction of skin and soft tissue defects is essential for good outcomes in the hand and upper extremity after trauma, cancer resection, or other indications. At the apex of the reconstructive ladder is microsurgical reconstruction through free-tissue transfer, which closes defects that cannot be achieved through less-arduous techniques, such as pedicled flaps, local tissue rearrangement, or skin grafts.

This special issue focuses on advances in techniques for microsurgical reconstruction. Some recent innovations include the use of ultrasound for preoperative flap planning and thinner flaps from better donor sites to create a more aesthetically pleasing reconstruction. Other techniques refine toe transfers, functional muscle transfers, and lymphedema surgery to achieve better patient outcomes.

An international cast of authors from Asia, Europe, and North and South America toiled to produce this issue to highlight the amazing work being done around the world in pushing the frontiers of what is possible in microsurgical reconstruction.

Harvey Chim, MD
Department of Surgery
University of Florida College of Medicine
Gainesville, FL 32610, USA

Kevin C. Chung, MD, MS
Michigan Medicine
University of Michigan
Comprehensive Hand Center
Ann Arbor, MI 48105, USA

E-mail addresses:
harveychim@yahoo.com (H. Chim)
kecchung@med.umich.edu (K.C. Chung)

Hand Clin 40 (2024) xiii
https://doi.org/10.1016/j.hcl.2024.02.001
0749-0712/24/© 2024 Published by Elsevier Inc.

hand.theclinics.com

Recent Advances in Upper Extremity Microsurgery
From Traditional to Perforator Flaps

Widya Adidharma, MD, Kevin C. Chung, MD, MS*

KEYWORDS

- Upper extremity reconstruction • Perforator flap • Profunda artery perforator flap
- Superficial circumflex iliac artery perforator flap

KEY POINTS

- The upper extremity has unique functional and aesthetic requirements. Reconstruction of upper extremity soft tissue defects should ideally provide coverage for vital structures, facilitate early mobilization, be thin and pliable to match its slim contour, and reestablish sensation.
- Perforator flaps such as the profunda artery perforator and superficial circumflex iliac artery perforator flaps can be raised on the superficial fascia, which creates a thin and pliable yet durable and supple flap option to match the contour and functional needs of the upper extremity.
- Comparisons to traditional reconstructive methods should be performed to assess whether these innovations in microsurgical reconstruction of upper extremity defects provide an improved functional and aesthetic benefit over traditional methods.

INTRODUCTION

There are several unique considerations that need to be made when reconstructing upper extremity defects. The upper extremity has several degrees of freedom that facilitate many complex movements needed for activities of daily living and for more intricate activities such as surgery and needlework. Our hands are also important for feeling and interacting with the world around us; specialized mechanoreceptors and thermoreceptors in our hands enable us to feel the warm touch of our child's hand and our hand gestures help to emphasize aspects of our conversation. Restoration of these important functional movements and sensations is a major goal in upper extremity reconstruction. Furthermore, as the upper extremity is exposed and plays a key role in social interactions, the reconstruction should have an aesthetic outcome.

Although skin grafting and locoregional flaps are commonly used to reconstruct minor upper extremity defects, reconstruction with free flaps is required for larger and more complex defects. Particularly when there is extensive soft tissue loss or there is exposure of vital structures (vessels, nerves, bones, and tendons), free flap reconstruction is desirable because free flaps transfer healthy tissue to an injured area, and the blood supply can improve bone healing and prevent infection.[1] Furthermore, skin grafting and locoregional flaps often prevent early mobilization. Skin grafts can lead to contractures, joint stiffness, pigmentation, and require a healthy wound bed, whereas free flaps are less likely to cause contractures and can restore volume deficits. Free flaps can also be performed in a single stage, which can improve postoperative rehabilitation and reduce hospitalization and health care expenditures.[2,3]

Given the functional requirements of the upper extremity, the reconstructive flap of choice should protect any vital structures, prevent excessive adhesion formation for underlying tendon gliding, and facilitate early mobilization through the joints.

Department of Surgery, Section of Plastic Surgery, University of Michigan Medical School, 1500 E. Medical Center Drive, 2130 Taubman Center, SPC 5340, Ann Arbor, MI 48109-5340, USA
* Corresponding author. Section of Plastic Surgery, The University of Michigan Health System, 1500 E. Medical Center Drive, 2130 Taubman Center, SPC 5340, Ann Arbor, MI 48109-5340.
E-mail address: kecchung@med.umich.edu

Hand Clin 40 (2024) 161–166
https://doi.org/10.1016/j.hcl.2023.08.006
0749-0712/24/© 2023 Elsevier Inc. All rights reserved.

For areas of heavy usage such as the hand, the reconstruction needs to be versatile. Finally, the chosen flap should also be thin and pliable to match the slim contour of the upper extremity. Given these considerations, fasciocutaneous flaps are often the ideal choice in upper extremity reconstruction. Compared to muscle flaps, fasciocutaneous flaps form less adhesions and therefore are better for tendon gliding and are easier to elevate again if needed. Traditional fasciocutaneous free flaps for the reconstruction of the upper extremity include the anterolateral thigh (ALT), radial forearm, lateral arm, and temporoparietal fascial free flaps.[4] When more bulk is needed, particularly for combined volar-dorsal defects in a through-and-through injury, muscle flaps can be helpful. Free muscle flaps that are often used in the upper extremity include the latissimus dorsi, rectus abdominis, and gracilis flaps. Though traditional free flaps play a major role in upper extremity reconstruction, they do not come without disadvantages. The thickness of raised fasciocutaneous free flaps is heavily influenced by the patient's body mass index (BMI) and the donor site region. If the raised flap is too thick, this will not match the thin skin and contour of the upper extremity. Furthermore, if the injury is extensive and a large flap needs to be raised, this results in a large donor defect and a sizable, reconstructed area that is insensate.

Fortunately, refinements in microsurgery techniques, more sophisticated flap planning, and improvements in understanding of the blood supply to various tissues around the body have led to an ongoing evolution of our reconstructive options and thus the ability to optimize both functional and aesthetic outcomes. This article will discuss more recent microsurgery innovations in upper extremity reconstruction toward the advancement of functional and aesthetic outcomes. This includes the use of newer perforator flaps, harvesting on the superficial fascia, and flap neurotization to restore sensation in upper extremity reconstruction.

THIN PERFORATOR FLAPS IN UPPER EXTREMITY RECONSTRUCTION

The discovery of the perforator flap has expanded the repertoire of free flaps that can be used in upper extremity reconstruction. Perforator flaps are perfused by an artery that perforates the deep muscle or fascia. In the 1990s, Allen and colleagues revolutionized autologous breast reconstruction by developing the deep inferior epigastric perforator (DIEP) flap technique as an alternative to the traditional transverse rectus abdominis musculocutaneous flap, thus preserving the rectus abdominis muscle and resulting in faster recovery.[5] The DIEP flap is considered the first perforator flap that was developed and widely recognized, and has paved the way for the development of other perforator flaps. By harvesting the flap on the perforator rather than the primary artery, microsurgeons can spare the underlying muscle and fascia, avoiding unnecessary donor site morbidity, healing complications, and prolonged recovery.

Furthermore, raising a flap on a perforator facilitates easier and safer thinning of flaps during the harvest. The blood supply of perforator flaps has a segmental vascularization pattern and therefore allows selective thinning of the flap without compromising the viability of the flap. Improvement in microsurgery techniques and understanding of soft tissue blood supply has enabled microsurgeons to combine the concept of flap thinning with perforator flap harvest to safely create thinner flaps that are more fitting for use in the upper extremity. A thin flap can be created by primary flap elevation on the superficial fascia (**Fig. 1**).[6] More recently, flap elevation on the "superthin" plane, flaps raised on the subdermal vascular network, has also been described.[7,8] Both the thin and superthin flaps can be performed at the time of harvest regardless of the BMI, which is advantageous for upper extremity reconstruction. Keeping a small thickness of fat protects underlying structures and hardware while matching the skin of the upper extremity. The ability to raise a flap on a perforator and thin a flap at the time of harvest expands the flap options that can be used in the upper extremity. Here, the authors will discuss 2 perforator flaps that were transformed for upper extremity reconstruction: thin profunda artery perforator (PAP) flaps and thin superficial circumflex iliac perforator (SCIP) flaps.

Profunda Artery Perforator Flap

The profunda artery perforator (PAP) flap has been well described in the literature for breast reconstruction. Studies have shown that the PAP flap has consistent perforators that can be found in

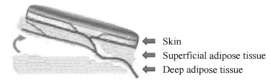

Fig. 1. Raising a thin free flap on the superficial fascial layer. (*Adapted from* **Fig. 1**B in Narushima, M., *et al.* Pure Skin Perforator Flaps: The Anatomical Vascularity of the Superthin Flap. *Plast Reconstr Surg* **142**, 351e–360e (2018).)

the posteromedial thigh and that there is reliable flap perfusion that can be based on a single perforator in that area.[9] It has a relatively large main flap artery caliber (average of 16 mm) as compared to many other flaps and long pedicle length (average of 6.8 cm), making it desirable for ease of identification during harvest and for reconstruction.[10] Aside from being a reliable flap, 1 of the major advantages of the PAP flap over many other flaps is the concealed donor site in the posteromedial thigh, which is not visible from the front and is hidden in the gluteal crease. Patients have found this to be more appealing than ALT flap reconstructions.[11]

Conventional PAP flaps have a desirable thickness for breast reconstruction but are too thick to use in upper extremity patients. This is particularly true for patients with a larger BMI as there is thick subcutaneous fat in the posteromedial thigh. Therefore, to transform the PAP flap into a more suitable option for upper extremity reconstruction, the flap should be thinned, which can be performed at the time of harvest. Thin PAP flaps are raised from anterior to posterior in the thin or superthin plane until 1 to 2 cm from the dominant perforator when the dissection is transitioned into the subfascial plane.[10] The dissection is carried proximally until enough perforator length is dissected at which point the dissection is continued posteriorly again in the thin or superthin plane to complete the harvest. In a case series of 10 patients, the mean flap thickness achieved was 0.7 cm, and the average surface size was 18.6 × 7.6 cm.[10] In this study, thin PAP flaps were used to reconstruct 3 upper extremity wounds and 7 lower extremity wounds. In the upper extremity, their flap success was 100%. In another case series of 28 patients by the same author, of which 9 reconstructions were in the upper extremity, there was no flap failure or flap necrosis in the upper extremity reconstructions and only minor complication of donor site superficial wound dehiscence.[12] There were no other reported outcomes other than these 2 case series. However, these case series do illustrate that thin PAP flaps can be harvested in the thin or superthin plane with reliable perfusion from a single dominant PAP perforator and can be used safely in upper extremity reconstruction.

Superficial Circumflex Iliac Artery Perforator Flap

Another example of a perforator flap that can be thinned and used in upper extremity reconstruction is the superficial circumflex iliac artery perforator (SCIP) flap. The SCIP flap was first described for extremity reconstruction by Koshima and colleagues in 2004.[13] Like the conventional groin flap, it is based off the superficial circumflex iliac artery (SCIA) system. Whereas the conventional groin flap uses the whole length of the of the SCIA system, the SCIP flap only requires a perforator. This facilitates flap thinning at the time of harvest, whereas a conventional groin flap that has thick fatty tissue should not be thinned aggressively as its blood supply runs subfascially or is in the fatty tissue deep layer.[13] When raised on the superficial fascia, the SCIP flap has a desirable thickness for finger and hand reconstruction cases. In a paper by Narushima and colleagues, thin SCIP flaps (**Fig. 2**) were raised on the superficial fascia with inclusion of a large subcutaneous vein for venous drainage and an intercostal nerve for sensory neurotization.[8] Six patients underwent finger and hand reconstruction with thin SCIP flaps, which were all less than or equal to 2 mm in thickness with a mean surface area of 46.3 cm^2. The mean perforator diameter was 0.8 mm and the mean pedicle length was 5.17 cm. All flaps survived with no necrosis, though 1 patient had venous congestion and required vein reanastomosis. In the 2 discussed cases, they noted that the patients were satisfied, and the reconstructions facilitated return to daily activities, though there was variable return of sensation as assessed by the Semmes-Weinstein test.

More recently, Ou and colleagues described the use of the SCIP flap for the reconstruction of multiple defects of the fingers and hand in a case series of 41 patients who underwent single-stage repair with either single or multi-lobed free SCIP flaps.[14] The superficial abdominal wall artery medial to the SCIA superficial branch can be used as the other vessel for a bilobed flap. Of the 41 patients, 3 had vascular compromise of the flaps, though they resolved with exploration and there was no flap loss. The reported outcomes had good aesthetic, functional, and sensory restoration and minimal complications and morbidity. Functionally, the patients had total active motion (TAM) test scores that were statistically similar as non-injured digits for each patient, and a normal range of pinch power as tested by the grasp and pinch power test. Excellent sensory recovery was also noted, which will be discussed in detail in the Neurotized Flaps section. The appearance of the flap and donor site outcomes were assessed with the Modified Vancouver Scar scale (MVSS), which is ranked from 0 to 15, where a lower score is better aesthetic appearance. In this study, the average MVSS was 1. It was also noted that the flaps were well matched in pigmentation and texture to the surrounding skin and there was no hypertrophy or erythema.

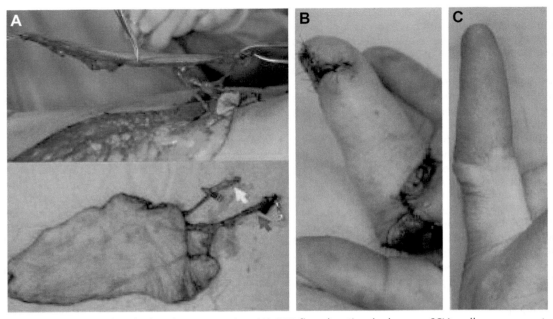

Fig. 2. Thin free SCIP flap for hand reconstruction. (*A*) SCIP flap elevation (red *arrow*: SCIA, yellow *arrow*: cutaneous vein), (*B*) SCIP flap coverage of a middle finger in the immediate postoperative period, (*C*) the reconstruction 1 year after operation. SCIA, superficial circumflex iliac artery; SCIP, superficial circumflex iliac artery perforator. (*Adapted from* Figs. 3A-B and Figure 2B & D Narushima, M., *et al.* Pure Skin Perforator Flaps: The Anatomical Vascularity of the Superthin Flap. *Plast Reconstr Surg* **142**, 351e-360e (2018)).

SCIP flaps do have several disadvantages. Most notably, SCIP flaps have a short pedicle, small vessel diameter, and inconsistent anatomy.[15] As a result of its variable anatomy and small vessel diameter, there is likely a steeper learning curve when using this flap. Nevertheless, the thin SCIP flap is a reasonable option for upper extremity reconstruction. The skin in the groin area is hairless and has similar texture and thickness as upper extremity skin, which makes it a good donor site for upper extremity reconstruction. Additionally, as compared to the conventional groin flap, the SCIP flap preserves the deep fascia, thus preventing hernia formation.

NEUROTIZED FLAPS

Our fingers are a specialized part of our body. The skin in our fingers house sensory organs that identify tactile and temperature sensations that enable interactions with our surrounding environment, detect painful stimuli that keep us safe from potential dangers, and play a role in modulation of complex and precise movements. Therefore, the reconstruction of fingers should incorporate the goal of sensory restoration. Free perforator flaps can often be harvested with cutaneous nerves, which could provide an advantage in sensory restoration compared to more traditional skin grafting or local flaps. For example, in thin SCIP flaps, the intercostal nerve can be harvested along with the flap for neurotization.[8] In the multi-lobed SCIP flap case series described by Ou and colleagues, the authors harvested the flaps with a cutaneous nerve and at 10.5 months, only 3 of 41 patients had mild hypoesthesia of the reconstructed area whereas the remaining patients had normal sensation over the flap on Semmes-Weinstein monofilament testing and no flap had loss of protective sensation.[14] Neurotized free composite ulnar artery perforator flaps from the volar wrist have also been described for the reconstruction of complex digital soft tissue defects. In a case series of 30 patients with defects of various volar and dorsal finger defects, the ulnar artery perforator flap was harvested with the medial antebrachial cutaneous nerve.[16] Interestingly, this could also be harvested with a part of the flexor carpi ulnaris to make a composite flap, which is advantageous as tissue is not harvested from multiple donor sites and the tissue is not separated from its original blood supply. The flap sensation recovery rate was excellent in 84% of the cases as assessed by 2-point discrimination and the hand sensory function criteria developed by the British Medical Research Association. Furthermore, the TAM scores of the affected digits demonstrated good return of finger function.

Flap neurotization has also benefited distal fingertip reconstruction. A newly described method is the neurotization of the hypothenar free perforator flap (HFPF). The HFPF was first described by Kim and colleagues in 2013 for the reconstruction of fingertip defects.[17] Dagdelen and colleagues then published a case series in 2020 of 12 patients who underwent HFPF with neural repair.[18] There was partial loss of the flap in 2 cases. There was return of sensation, though expectedly less than non-operated fingers as assessed by dynamic and static 2-point discrimination tests. The overall satisfaction in the Michigan Hand Outcomes Questionnaire was 92.7%. Unfortunately, there was no comparison to other fingertip treatment strategies such as semi-occlusive dressing therapy, which has shown better subjective aesthetics and reduced loss of 2-point discrimination compared to patients who underwent surgery.[19]

LIMITATIONS AND FUTURE DIRECTIONS

Although the discussed microsurgical advances have resulted in both functional and aesthetic reconstructions of the upper extremity, there are several important considerations to point out. Most of the discussed articles were case series without comparisons to more traditional reconstructive options. For example, for the SCIP flap in finger reconstruction, the studies demonstrated good aesthetic, functional, and sensory restoration; however, there were no comparisons in functional and aesthetic restoration to skin grafts, local flaps, regional flaps, and traditional free flap reconstruction. More rigorous outcome studies could shed light on whether these reconstructive options provide significantly improved sensory and functional outcomes compared to traditional methods.

It should also be noted that these techniques imply longer learning curves, more experience, and potentially more resources. Harvesting a flap on a perforator and thinning a perforator add additional microsurgical challenges. Furthermore, many of the case series used advanced imaging for preoperative perforator mapping to help with efficiency in perforator flap elevation and thinning the flaps. For example, in 1 PAP flap approach, computed tomography angiography is used to localize the dominant perforator followed by characterizing the suprafascial branching pattern of the perforator using a color Doppler ultrasound, which aids in efficient dissection and customization of the flap for extremity reconstruction.[12] Another study used indocyanine green angiography to confirm perfusion of the flap.[8] Whether these imaging techniques are needed in every reconstruction is unclear and is likely dependent on the training, expertise, and/or choice of the surgeon. Though this could increase resource utilization, it is evident that advanced imaging has helped our understanding of the anatomy and blood supply of tissue and development in microsurgery innovations.

SUMMARY

Refinements in microsurgery techniques, more sophisticated flap planning, and improvements in understanding of tissue blood supply have led to the development of perforator flaps that better suit the functional and aesthetic needs of upper extremity reconstruction. Newer perforator flaps such as the thin PAP and thin SCIP flaps minimize donor site morbidity and visibility, can be raised on the thin or superthin plane to match the slimmer contour of the upper extremity, and can be neurotized to restore sensation. Though further studies are needed to elucidate the functional and aesthetic outcomes of these newer flaps and to compare the outcomes to more traditional flaps, these innovations do expand the free flap repertoire of upper extremity reconstructive options and push the boundaries of reconstructive microsurgery in the upper extremity.

CLINICS CARE POINTS

- The upper extremity has unique functional and aesthetic requirements. Reconstruction of upper extremity soft tissue defects should ideally provide coverage for vital structures, facilitate early mobilization, be thin and pliable to match its slimmer contour, and reestablish sensation.

- Perforator flaps such as the PAP and SCIP flaps can be raised on the superficial fascia, which creates a thin and pliable yet durable and supple flap option to match the contour and functional needs of the upper extremity.

- Comparisons to traditional reconstructive methods should be performed to assess whether these innovations in microsurgical reconstruction of upper extremity defects provide an improved functional and aesthetic benefit over traditional methods.

DISCLOSURE

Dr K.C. Chung receives funding from the National Institutes of Health, United States and book royalties from Wolters Kluwer and Elsevier.

FUNDING

None.

REFERENCES

1. Herter F, Ninkovic M, Ninkovic M. Rational flap selection and timing for coverage of complex upper extremity trauma. J Plast Reconstr Aesthet Surg 2007;60(7):760–8.

2. King EA, Ozer K. Free skin flap coverage of the upper extremity. Hand Clin 2014;30(2):201–9, vi.

3. Chim H, Ng ZY, Carlsen BT, et al. Soft tissue coverage of the upper extremity: an overview. Hand Clin 2014;30(4):459–73, vi.

4. Pederson WC. Upper extremity microsurgery. Plast Reconstr Surg 2001;107(6):1524–37 [discussion: 1538-9, 1540-3].

5. Allen RJ, Treece P. Deep inferior epigastric perforator flap for breast reconstruction. Ann Plast Surg 1994;32(1):32–8.

6. Hong JP, Choi DH, Suh H, et al. A new plane of elevation: the superficial fascial plane for perforator flap elevation. J Reconstr Microsurg 2014;30(7):491–6.

7. Chin T, Ogawa R, Murakami M, et al. An anatomical study and clinical cases of 'super-thin flaps' with transverse cervical perforator. Br J Plast Surg 2005;58(4):550–5.

8. Narushima M, Yamasoba T, Iida T, et al. Pure Skin Perforator Flaps: The Anatomical Vascularity of the Superthin Flap. Plast Reconstr Surg 2018;142(3): 351e–60e.

9. Largo RD, Chu CK, Chang EI, et al. Perforator Mapping of the Profunda Artery Perforator Flap: Anatomy and Clinical Experience. Plast Reconstr Surg 2020; 146(5):1135–45.

10. Chim H. The Superthin Profunda Artery Perforator Flap for Extremity Reconstruction: Clinical Implications. Plast Reconstr Surg 2022;150(4):915–8.

11. Wu JC, Huang JJ, Tsao CK, et al. Comparison of Posteromedial Thigh Profunda Artery Perforator Flap and Anterolateral Thigh Perforator Flap for Head and Neck Reconstruction. Plast Reconstr Surg 2016;137(1):257–66.

12. Chim H. Perforator mapping and clinical experience with the superthin profunda artery perforator flap for reconstruction in the upper and lower extremities. J Plast Reconstr Aesthet Surg 2023;81:60–7.

13. Koshima I, Nanba Y, Tsutsui T, et al. Superficial circumflex iliac artery perforator flap for reconstruction of limb defects. Plast Reconstr Surg 2004; 113(1):233–40.

14. Ou CL, Li J, Zhou X, et al. Repair of multiple hand defects with superficial circumflex iliac artery perforator flap. Injury 2023;54(3):940–6.

15. Tashiro K, Yamashita S. Superficial Circumflex Iliac Artery Perforator Flap for Dorsalis Pedis Reconstruction. Plast Reconstr Surg Glob Open 2017;5(4): e1308.

16. Qi JW, Ding MC, Zhang H, et al. Repair of complex digital soft-tissue defects using a free composite ulnar artery perforator flap from the volar wrist. Int Wound J 2023;20(5):1678–86.

17. Kim KS, Kim ES, Hwang JH, et al. Fingertip reconstruction using the hypothenar perforator free flap. J Plast Reconstr Aesthet Surg 2013;66(9):1263–70.

18. Dagdelen D, Aksoy A. Evaluation of neurotized hypothenar free perforator flaps used for fingertip reconstruction. Ann Plast Surg 2020;84(2):e1–6.

19. Pastor T, Hermann P, Haug L, et al. Semi-occlusive dressing therapy versus surgical treatment in fingertip amputation injuries: a clinical study. Eur J Trauma Emerg Surg 2023;49(3):1441–7.

Evolution and Application of Ultrasound for Flap Planning in Upper Extremity Reconstruction

Ramin Shekouhi, MD, Harvey Chim, MD*

KEYWORDS

- Flap planning • Ultrasound • Color Doppler ultrasound • Computed tomography angiography
- Magnetic resonance angiography

KEY POINTS

- Compared with handheld doppler, ultrasound has considerable advantages for preoperative flap planning including mapping and assessment of perforator location and anatomy.
- Although computed tomography angiography (CTA) is the most common imaging modality used for flap planning in the trunk, color Doppler ultrasound (CDU) has a number of advantages in the extremities due to anatomic differences.
- Disadvantages of CTA for flap planning include the requirement for radiation exposure, contrast agent administration, and its high cost.
- CDU is a more cost-effective imaging modality with excellent sensitivity and specificity for perforator mapping in the extremities.

INTRODUCTION

The key to the success of perforator flaps is the accurate preoperative localization of dominant perforators. Preoperative perforator mapping can minimize the difficulties with intraoperative localization of perforators as well as partial or complete flap loss related to disturbed blood flow and inadequate perfusion.[1,2] With preoperative information regarding the trajectory, diameter, and anatomic positioning of the perforators, flap design can be optimized, the duration of the surgical procedure reduced, flap survival improved, and postoperative complications decreased. The most common imaging modalities used preoperatively for flap planning are computed tomography angiography (CTA), magnetic resonance angiography (MRA), and ultrasound (US).[3–5]

The ideal imaging modality is the one that can provide reproducible accurate information regarding the location of the perforator while being cost-effective, easily accessible, and reducing exposure to radiation.[6] Numerous studies have advocated CTA as the preferred option for preoperative flap planning,[7–9] whereas more recently color Doppler ultrasound (CDU) has become popular.[3,10] We review the current literature on the application of various imaging modalities for flap planning, with a focus on the application of US as a tool for preoperative perforator mapping.

HISTORY OF ULTRASOUND FOR FLAP PLANNING

Initial case reports described the use of US for the monitoring of a buried free fibular flap[11] and the localization of recipient vessels for free tissue transfer.[12] Subsequently Amerhauser and colleagues[13] in 1993 studied the efficacy of CDU as a microvascular assessment technique in animal

Division of Plastic & Reconstructive Surgery, Department of Surgery, University of Florida College of Medicine, 1600 Southwest Archer Road, Gainesville, FL32610, USA
* Corresponding author.
E-mail address: harveychim@yahoo.com

Hand Clin 40 (2024) 167–177
https://doi.org/10.1016/j.hcl.2023.08.007

models and found that this was effective for assessing venous and arterial occlusion and insufficiency, preoperatively and postoperatively.[13]

In 1994, Hallock and colleagues[14] studied the accuracy of CDU as a preoperative assessment tool for evaluating dominant perforators perfusing fasciocutaneous flaps. They showed that preoperative CDU can objectively identify cutaneous perforators with high sensitivity and specificity, which laid the foundation for employing CDU in the field of reconstructive microsurgery.[14,15] Building upon this research, Cheng and colleagues[16] reported that preoperative Doppler assessment can reduce the risk of partial flap necrosis in patients undergoing a pedicled posterior interosseous artery flap. It has been shown that compared with other US modes, CDU provides enhanced direct visualization of microvessels as small as 0.2 mm, along with the ability to map their suprafascial course and perivascular anatomy.[12,17]

In 1994, Rand and colleagues[18] were one of the firsts to assess the efficacy of CDU for preoperative transverse rectus abdominis myocutaneous (TRAM) flap planning. Their findings demonstrated that the identification of the dominant perforator using CDU can substantially improve flap survival.[18] Berg and colleagues also showed that CDU is an accurate imaging modality for designing TRAM flaps, which can greatly enhance flap survival and minimize the duration of the surgical procedure.[19] Blondeel and colleagues subsequently assessed the sensitivity and predictive value of preoperative CDU for deep inferior epigastric perforator (DIEP) flap planning compared with results of unidirectional Doppler flowmetry.[20] They observed an unfavorable incidence of false negatives associated with unidirectional Doppler flowmetry, leading them to recommend intraoperative CDU as the preferred choice for flap planning.[20] Another study showed that preoperative CDU was useful for localizing the perforating vessels for flaps in the lower abdominal wall or buttock for breast reconstruction within 0.8 cm.[21]

For other flaps, Futran and colleagues[22] reported the efficacy of CDU for evaluating the peroneal vessels as well as collateral circulation in candidates for fibular flaps. Compared to CTA and MRA, CDU was found be comparable in accuracy, with lower cost and no morbidity.[22] CDU was also used to evaluate alterations in flow patterns in the forearm after the harvest of a radial forearm flap, with findings that another axis based on the anterior interosseous artery develops, maintaining global arterial inflow to the hand.[23]

Specific to the upper extremity, Frost-Arner and colleagues reported that CDU can effectively identify dominant perforators for local flap reconstruction

in the elbow.[24] Other studies have further reinforced the efficacy of CDU for local and free flap reconstruction in the hand and upper extremity, reducing the incidence of partial flap necrosis and increasing overall flap survival.[25,26]

OTHER IMAGING MODALITIES
Handheld Doppler

Handheld Doppler (HHD) uses high-frequency sound waves to assess vessels beneath the skin. Once the sound waves encounter an artery or a vein, they are detected by the transducer, creating echoes that are then converted into audible signals.[27] High-pitched sounds, often characterized as a "whooshing" sound, indicate blood flow moving toward the transducer. Conversely, lower pitched sounds signify reverse blood flow.[28] Advantages of HHD include easy portability, low cost, and its noninvasive nature.

The main disadvantage of HHD for perforator detection is its high false-positive rate.[29] It has been speculated that the reason for this high false-positive rate is the pickup of signals from adjacent axial vessels, which can be misinterpreted as perforators. Therefore, a signal detected using HHD may not accurately correspond to the actual location of a perforator.[4] Also, HHD falls short in detecting the exact course of a perforating vessel for flap harvest.[30] Additionally, HHD is only capable of detecting perforators that do not exceed the depth of 20 mm. As such, HHD is not able to map the deep or subfascial course of a perforator. When harvesting flaps in a subfascial plane, the signal detected using HHD may not necessarily correspond to the true location of the perforator. Finally, the loudness of the audible signal on HHD may not necessarily correspond with the size or caliber of the perforator. Ideally, when choosing a perforator to base a flap on, the largest sized perforator would be used. Thus, these limitations need to be considered when using HHD in preoperative flap planning.

Computed Tomography Angiography

CTA is the most commonly used imaging modality for preoperative flap planning due to its capacity for high-resolution visualization of perforators and 3-dimensional reconstruction.[31] Disadvantages compared to CDU include the requirement for radiation exposure and contrast administration, both of which carry potential risks including radiation-induced tissue damage and renal insufficiency.[4] In addition, CTA provides static images acquired during the scan, whereas CDU gives real-time assessment of blood flow and dynamic evaluation of vascular structures. This real-time information can be valuable for assessing vessel patency and flow dynamics.[3,32] In addition, CTA is generally more expensive than CDU and may have limited availability in some hospital settings.[3]

CTA is generally considered the preferred option for preoperative flap planning in the abdomen.[33,34] However, CDU may be a more suitable option for extremities due to anatomic differences including the lack of thick subcutaneous tissue and their tubular structure. Accordingly, in regions with thicker adipose tissue like the abdominal cavity, CTA offers superior visualization of perforators. While CDU is unable to provide a distinct blood flow signal in deeper tissue layers due to intermittent image capture, it demonstrates high sensitivity in detecting perforators within superficial tissue planes where hemodynamic signals are more easily identifiable.[3,10,35,36]

Combination approaches for the use of CTA and CDU have been advocated to acquire further detailed information about the exact location and course of perforators for planning of thin profunda artery perforator (PAP) flaps. In this approach, the location of the dominant perforator can be accurately located using CTA, followed by utilization of CDU to visualize the course and precise anatomy of the vessels.[37]

Magnetic Resonance Angiography

Unlike radiation-based imaging techniques, MRA utilizes non-iodine contrast agents, making it a safer procedure. It generates a 3-dimensional image, enabling surgeons to accurately evaluate the path and size of blood perforators and the adjacent structures.[38,39] Additionally, MRA can be obtained in both prone and supine positions, ensuring that images preserve the natural tissue contours without any distortion caused by pressure against a flat surface. Some drawbacks associated with MRA include its relatively high cost. Moreover, its use is limited in claustrophobic patients or patients with metal implants.[40] MRA has been commonly utilized for preoperative planning of free fibula flaps.

MRA is preferred over CTA by some authors for visualizing the vascular anatomy in preoperative planning for DIEP flaps.[41] The current literature lacks sufficient data regarding the comparison of the sensitivity and specificity of MRA and CDU. Nevertheless, CDU offers advantages over MRA in terms of portability and widespread availability as well as cost-effectiveness, allowing for bedside evaluation.

COLOR DOPPLER ULTRASOUND- TECHNICAL CONSIDERATIONS

Brightness mode (B-mode) is the basic imaging mode of the US device, which provides a 2-dimensional gray scale image of the underlying anatomy. Typically, the first step for perforator mapping is to evaluate the structural anatomy of the targeted location using the B-mode. The skin is the most superficial layer indicated by a distinct, bright hyperechoic line on the US image, followed by the subcutaneous adipose layer which appears isoechoic. The muscle layer can be found deeper surrounded by the muscular fascia, which is commonly seen as a hyperechoic line in CDU.[4]

The color Doppler mode is most useful for the mapping of perforators and works by sending high-frequency signals to the underlying vessels, which cause a frequency shift when encountered with the moving red blood cells. The Doppler-shifted frequencies are then detected by the transducer and create a color-coded representation of the underlying blood flow.[42] When the blood flow is moving toward the probe, it is commonly represented by a red color. In contrast, when blood is flowing away from the transducer, it is typically represented as shades of blue. In general, locating the ideal perforator using CDU is a quick and straightforward procedure, with a reported median time of 3 minutes for the procedure.[43]

In our institution, the surgical team performs US examination on the operating table prior to surgery. The conventional US machine used by the anesthesia team is sufficient to localize the dominant perforator. In the initial phase of the learning curve, the focus should be on locating perforators, and more detailed mapping of the course of the perforator can be performed with increasing use and familiarity with the US machine. In our setting, routine mapping of perforators preoperatively takes about 5 to 10 minutes.

The color box is the rectangular area on the US display that represents the region of interest where blood flow is being assessed. In the color box, the color Doppler information is superimposed onto the B-mode image with different colors demonstrating the blood flow direction and velocity.[44] To achieve a maximized frame rate, a small color box should be selected. Then, with color Doppler mode, the perforator can be located by moving and tilting the US probe distally and proximally until an optimal image of the perforator is seen. The course of the perforator from the deep fascia heading suprafascial to the skin can be mapped and followed.

The flow velocity is represented by the color intensity (gain) which can be adjusted to maximize visualization. For low-velocity blood flow, adjusting pulse repetition frequency (PRF) to correlate to decreased blood flow can also improve visualization.[45] Initially, it is recommended to use the lowest PRF possible to visualize low-flow microvasculature and then increase the PRF to reach the threshold of the perforator flow velocity.[46]

Compared with the HHD, CDU has considerable advantages including comprehensive assessment of perforator anatomy, caliber, and flow velocity. In addition, CDU can be integrated with traditional grayscale US imaging, which can allow for simultaneous evaluation of structural anatomy and blood flow.[47] Furthermore, CDU offers additional Doppler modes, including power Doppler. This mode can provide detailed information about small perforators that may not be adequately visualized with standard CDU settings.[48]

Power Doppler ultrasonography (PDU) displays the amplitude of the Doppler signal in color rather than the velocity and direction of flow and hence enhances sensitivity to low-flow states, allowing for improved detection and evaluation of subtle blood flow in smaller vessels.[49] Kehrer and colleagues,[50] reported an excellent sensitivity of PDU for accurately identifying the location and musculocutaneous course of the perforators during PAP flap preoperative planning. However, it should be taken into consideration that PDU can potentially overestimate the size of perforators.[50] The observed disparity in size estimation is thought to arise from PDU's inability to distinguish flow direction within arteries and veins. This limitation necessitates adjustments in velocity and color scales, leading to an overestimation in perforator diameter.[50] Notably, this discrepancy has been widely reported for other imaging modalities, particularly for CTA.[51]

Additionally, US settings can be modified to enhance visualization of low-flow blood vessels, such as small perforators. One example is adjusting the wall filter, which helps eliminate vascular wall motion that improves blood flow visualization in small perforators.[47]

Nanno and colleagues[52] showed that CDU is a reliable option for preoperative planning of dorsal metacarpal artery perforator flaps. They reported a sensitivity rate of 100% and 95% for detection of the proximal and distal perforators, respectively. Compared with HHD, CDU was a superior option for detecting the cutaneous perforators in the upper extremity.[52] Wang and colleagues[53] reported that identification of the distribution and course of the dorsal digital artery perforators for flap planning was effectively achieved in all patients using CDU.[53] Preoperative CDU of the thoracodorsal pedicle was also found to improve the outcomes of latissimus dorsi flaps by assessing the patency of the pedicle preoperatively.[54]

For perforators with considerable anatomic variation, CDU has proven to be highly reliable when it comes to flap planning. According to a study by Tashiro and colleagues,[55] CDU exhibited a sensitivity rate of 100% in accurately identifying perforators of the thoracodorsal artery when elevating a thoracodorsal artery perforator flap. Additionally, CDU has shown favorable outcomes in the preoperative planning of PAP flaps elevated in the thin or superthin plane.[37,56]

When flaps are elevated in a suprafascial or thinner plane, preoperative localization of perforators is crucial. This allows rapid and safe elevation of the flap away from the perforator, reducing operative time.[57] This reduces the need for flap thinning in contrast to flaps elevated in a traditional subfascial plane.

HIGH AND ULTRAHIGH FREQUENCY ULTRASOUND

High-frequency ultrasound (HFUS) refers to US settings with frequencies more than 20 MHz. Compared to conventional US, there is improved resolution, better visualization of small vessels and superficial structures,[58] and superior sensitivity in detecting low-velocity blood flow (**Fig. 1**). HFUS has been used for the diagnosis of skin-related disorders due to its ability to differentiate superficial structures smaller than 100 μm.[59] More recently HFUS has become popular for preoperative flap planning. A study by Gong and colleagues[60] reported the efficacy of HFUS in preoperative planning of myocutaneous fibular flaps, with a sensitivity of 89.4%, specificity of 78.6%, and accuracy of 85.3%.[60]

HFUS has shown to an effective assessment tool for anterolateral thigh (ALT) flap planning with a sensitivity rate of 94.7%.[61] HFUS has the capability to provide a precise and detailed visualization of the primary perforators, along with their spatial correlation to the adjacent anatomic structures which can potentially lead to enhanced flap survival.[62] Incorporating HFUS into preoperative flap assessment also allows for optimal identification of the type and distribution of dorsal digital artery perforators.[53] Additionally, reports regarding the use of ultrahigh frequency US for preoperative planning of superficial circumflex iliac artery perforator (SCIP) flaps have shown promising results, demonstrating favorable outcomes in terms of flap viability.[63,64]

Specific to the SCIP flap, which is perfused in an axial fashion throughout its course, the location and caliber of the pedicle, which is superficial, can be very accurately assessed using ultrahigh frequency US and HFUS. Unlike other perforator flaps, assessment of deeper vessels is not required, and hence depth limitations inherent to the use of ultrahigh frequency US and HFUS are not an issue.

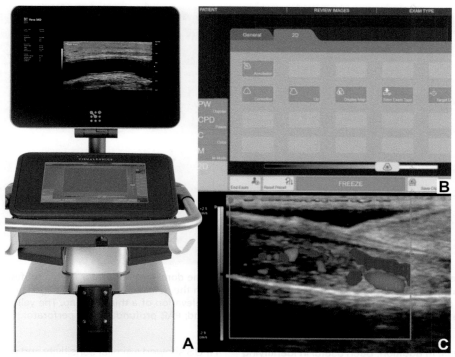

Fig. 1. (*A*, *B*) HFUS device and display. HFUS offers adjustable settings for depth, frequency, and gain for evaluating perforator vessels. (*C*) HFUS allows precise localization and course of small vessels under the nail bed. HFUS, high-frequency ultrasound (HFUS Vevo® MD, courtesy of FujiFilm VisualSonics, Inc.)

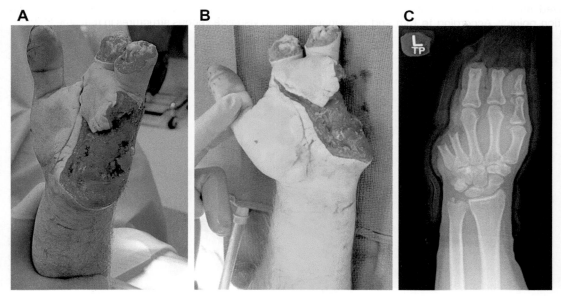

Fig. 2. Case 1. (*A*, *B*) A 24-year-old man sustained traumatic amputation of the left long and index fingers through the proximal interphalangeal (PIP) joint, amputation of the left ring and small fingers through the metacarpals, and a severe ulnar hand soft tissue defect. (*C*) Radiograph showing bony injuries.

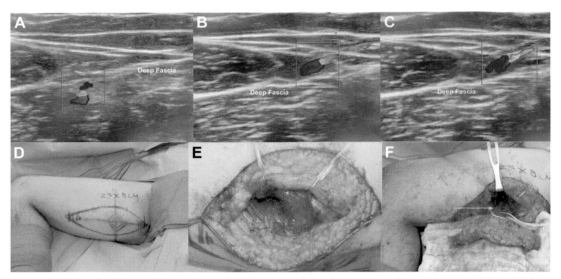

Fig. 3. Case 1. (*A–C*) Sequential CDU images follow course of the dominant perforator from a subfascial (*A*) to a suprafascial plane (*B, C*). (*D*) Design of the PAP flap centered on the dominant perforator imaged preoperatively with CDU. (*E*) Exposure of the dominant perforator. (*F*) After elevation of a thin PAP flap. The yellow arrow indicates the dominant perforator. CDU, color Doppler ultrasound; PAP, profunda artery perforator.

HFUS has, in addition, been useful in identifying functional lymphatic vessels prior to lymphovenous anastomosis for the treatment of refractory lymphedema.[65] The main challenge for preoperative lymphatic identification is to distinguish the lymphatic vessels from superficial veins. This can be accomplished by visualizing the lymphatic vessels that do not collapse when the probe pressure is increased.[66] Also, augmented flow can be visualized after massaging the distal end of the examination point.[67] According to Kim and colleagues,[67]

HFUS showed a similar sensitivity and positive predictive value in detecting viable lymphatic vessels at early stages of lymphedema when compared to commonly used imaging modalities for preoperative lymphatic detection, including indocyanine green lymphography and magnetic resonance lymphangiography.[67] However, at more advanced stages of lymphedema, HFUS showed statistically significant superiority in the identification of functional lymphatic vessels, as well as the capability to visualize venous structures in real time.[67]

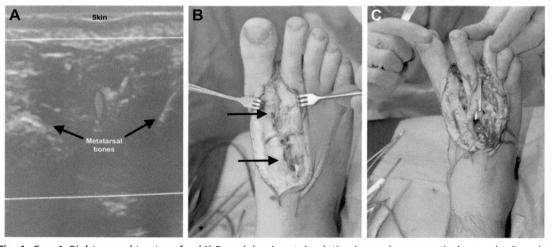

Fig. 4. Case 1. Right second toe transfer. (*A*) Dorsal dominant circulation imaged preoperatively on color Doppler ultrasound (CDU). (*B*) Dorsal dominant circulation (*arrows*) demonstrated intraoperatively. (*C*) After elevation of right second toe flap.

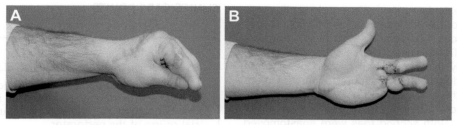

Fig. 5. Postoperative result after completion of reconstruction. (*A*) Lateral; (*B*) Palmar views.

CASE EXAMPLES ILLUSTRATING THE USE OF COLOR DOPPLER ULTRASOUND FOR PREOPERATIVE FLAP PLANNING
Case 1. Free Profunda Artery Perforator Flap with Bilateral Second Toe to Finger Transfer for Hand Reconstruction

A 24-year-old male presented after he sustained an injury to the left hand caused by a boat propeller (**Fig. 2**). Injuries included amputation of the left long and index fingers through the proximal interphalangeal joint, amputation of the left ring and small fingers through the metacarpals, and an ulnar hand soft tissue defect. The reconstructive plan consisted of 2 stages: (1) coverage of the ulnar hand defect and index and middle tip defects with a thin PAP flap to maintain the width of the palm and (2) reconstruction of the index and middle fingers with toe transfer to restore the tripod pinch.

In this case, the CDU was used for preoperative planning in both stages of the reconstruction. In the first stage, CDU was used in combination with CTA preoperatively to map the dominant perforator (**Fig. 3**A–C). This allowed precise design and elevation of a thin PAP flap for soft tissue coverage (**Fig. 3**D–F).

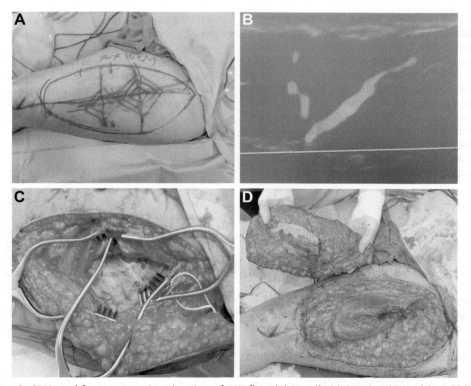

Fig. 6. Case 2. CDU used for preoperative planning of ALT flap. (*A*) Handheld doppler showed 2 audible signals. (*B*) CDU showed a sizable perforator only for the proximal signal. (*C*) Intraoperative exploration showed a branching pattern of the dominant perforator corresponding to preoperative CDU imaging. (*D*) Following elevation of a single perforator ALT flap in the thin plane. ALT, anterolateral thigh; CDU, color Doppler ultrasound.

Two weeks later, the patient underwent reconstruction of the left index and middle fingers with simultaneous bilateral second-toe transfers (**Fig. 4**). CDU was used to assess the pedicles preoperatively. In this case, both second toes showed a dorsal dominant circulation. Preoperative mapping of the pedicles allowed rapid harvest of both second toes using a proximal to distal approach. Both second toes were anastomosed to the dorsal radial artery on a common pedicle. The patient subsequently underwent staged surgery for division of flap syndactyly followed by further debulking and refinement. **Fig. 5** shows results 8.5 months after the first surgery, with functional tripod pinch.

Case 2. Anterolateral Thigh Free Flap

A 29-year-old female patient with a fourth-degree burn to the left dorsal foot after a candle fell over her while she was sleeping. She underwent multiple rounds of wound debridement by the burns team, following which she was referred for flap coverage. In this case, a free ALT flap was planned. HHD showed 2 areas with an audible signal (**Fig. 6**A). Upon imaging with the CDU (**Fig. 6**B), however, only the proximal site showed a sizable perforator which could be followed from a subfascial to a suprafascial plane. Intraoperative exploration (**Fig. 6**C) showed a branching pattern of the dominant perforator corresponding to preoperative CDU. This allowed rapid and safe elevation of a thin single perforator ALT flap harvested mostly in the suprascarpal plane (**Fig. 6**D). This case illustrates the accuracy of preoperative CDU compared to HHD for localizing and characterizing the dominant perforator, particularly useful when an ALT flap is elevated in the suprafascial, thin, or superthin planes.

SUMMARY

Accurate preoperative mapping of perforators facilitates rapid and safe elevation of free and pedicled fasciocutaneous flaps. US has a number of advantages compared with HHD. Compared with HHD, CDU offers great visibility of perforators while being inexpensive and widely available in hospital settings. Compared with CTA in the extremities, CDU may be advantageous due to the necessity of imaging more superficial vessels and the lack of thick subcutaneous tissue. Further advantages of CDU include the absence of radiation exposure and the nonnecessity for contrast agent administration, along with a real-time assessment of anatomic structures at the targeted location.

CLINICS CARE POINTS

- US is effective for preoperative flap planning.
- Color Doppler mode allows for the localization of the dominant perforator as well as the mapping of the subfascial and suprafascial course of the perforator.
- Power Doppler mode can be used to better assess small vessels.
- Applications of US in the hand and upper extremity include preoperative planning of free and pedicled perforator flaps as well as mapping of axial vessels where there is concern for anatomic variation.

DISCLOSURES

The authors have no conflict of interest and no financial interest in the discussed manuscript. No funding was received for this article.

REFERENCES

1. Khouri RK. Avoiding free flap failure. Clin Plast Surg 1992;19(4):773–81.
2. Yu P, Chang DW, Miller MJ, et al. Analysis of 49 cases of flap compromise in 1310 free flaps for head and neck reconstruction. Head Neck 2009;31(1):45–51.
3. Feng S, Min P, Grassetti L, et al. A prospective head-to-head comparison of color Doppler ultrasound and computed tomographic angiography in the preoperative planning of lower extremity perforator flaps. Plast Reconstr Surg 2016;137(1):335–47.
4. Chim H, Nichols DS, Chopan M. Ultrasound for Perforator Mapping and Flap Design in the Hand and Upper Extremity. J Hand Surg Am 2023;48(6):595–601.
5. Steenbeek LM, Peperkamp K, Ulrich DJ, et al. Alternative imaging technologies for perforator mapping in free flap breast reconstructive surgery–a comprehensive overview of the current literature. J Plast Reconstr Aesthetic Surg 2022;75(11):4074–84.
6. Rozen WM, Garcia-Tutor E, Alonso-Burgos A, et al. Planning and optimising DIEP flaps with virtual surgery: the Navarra experience. J J Plast Reconstr Aesthet Surg 2010;63(2):289–97.
7. Pratt GF, Rozen WM, Chubb D, et al. Preoperative imaging for perforator flaps in reconstructive surgery: a systematic review of the evidence for current techniques. Ann Plast Surg 2012;69(1):3–9.
8. Malhotra A, Chhaya N, Nsiah-Sarbeng P, et al. CT-guided deep inferior epigastric perforator (DIEP) flap localization—better for the patient, the surgeon, and the hospital. Clin Radiol 2013;68(2):131–8.

9. Ngaage LM, Hamed R, Oni G, et al. The role of CT angiography in assessing deep inferior epigastric perforator flap patency in patients with pre-existing abdominal scars. J Surg Res 2019;235:58–65.

10. Su W, Lu L, Lazzeri D, et al. Contrast-enhanced ultrasound combined with three-dimensional reconstruction in preoperative perforator flap planning. Plast Reconstr Surg 2013;131(1):80–93.

11. Stevenson TR, Rubin JM, Herzenberg JE. Vascular patency of fibular free graft: assessment by Doppler color-flow imager: a case report. J Reconstr Microsurg 1988;4(5):409–13.

12. Hutchinson DT. Color duplex imaging. Applications to upper-extremity and microvascular surgery. Hand Clin 1993;9(1):47–57.

13. Amerhauser A, Moelleken BR, Mathes SJ, et al. Color flow ultrasound for delineating microsurgical vessels: a clinical and experimental study. Ann Plast Surg 1993;30(3):193–203.

14. Hallock GG. Evaluation of fasciocutaneous perforators using color duplex imaging. Plast Reconstr Surg 1994;94(5):644–51.

15. Hallock GG. Color duplex imaging for identifying perforators prior to pretransfer expansion of fasciocutaneous free flaps. Ann Plast Surg 1994;32(6):595–601.

16. Cheng M-H, Chen H-C, Santamaria E, et al. Preoperative ultrasound Doppler study and clinical correlation of free posterior interosseous flap. Changgeng yi xue za zhi 1997;20(4):258–64.

17. Cheng H-T, Lin F-Y, Chang SC-N. Diagnostic efficacy of color Doppler ultrasonography in preoperative assessment of anterolateral thigh flap cutaneous perforators: an evidence-based review. Plast Reconstr Surg 2013;131(3):471e–3e.

18. Rand RP, Cramer MM, Strandness ED Jr. Color-flow duplex scanning in the preoperative assessment of TRAM flap perforators: a report of 32 consecutive patients. Plast Reconstr Surg 1994;93(3):453–9.

19. Berg WA, Chang BW, DeJong MR, et al. Color Doppler flow mapping of abdominal wall perforating arteries for transverse rectus abdominis myocutaneous flap in breast reconstruction: method and preliminary results. Radiology 1994;192(2):447–50.

20. Blondeel PN, Beyens G, Verhaeghe R, et al. Doppler flowmetry in the planning of perforator flaps. Br J Plast Surg 1998;51(3):202–9.

21. Giunta R, Geisweid A, Feller A. The value of preoperative Doppler sonography for planning free perforator flaps. Plast Reconstr Surg 2000;105(7):2381–6.

22. Futran ND, Stack BC, Payne LP. Use of color Doppler flow imaging for preoperative assessment in fibular osteoseptocutaneous free tissue transfer. Otolaryngol Head Neck Surg 1997;117(6):660–3.

23. Ciria-Llorens G, Gomez-Cia T, Talegon-Melendez A. Analysis of flow changes in forearm arteries after raising the radial forearm flap: a prospective study using colour duplex imaging. Br J Plast Surg 1999;52(6):440–4.

24. Frost–Arner L, Björgell O. Local perforator flap for reconstruction of deep tissue defects in the elbow area. Ann Plast Surg 2003;50(5):491–7.

25. Innocenti M, Baldrighi C, Delcroix L, et al. Local perforator flaps in soft tissue reconstruction of the upper limb. Handchir Mikrochir Plast Chir 2009;41(06):315–21.

26. Shen X-q, Shen H, Xu J-h, et al. Color Doppler imaging of an ulnar artery perforator forearm flap for resurfacing finger defects. Ann Plast Surg 2014;73(1):43–5.

27. Thrush A, Hartshorne T, Deane CR. Vascular ultrasound E-book: How, Why and when. Elsevier Health Sciences; 2021.

28. Nelson T, Pretorius D. The Doppler signal: where does it come from and what does it mean? AJR Am J Roentgenol 1988;151(3):439–47.

29. Khan UD, Miller J. Reliability of handheld Doppler in planning local perforator–based flaps for extremities. Aesthetic Plast Surg 2007;31:521–5.

30. Taylor GI, Doyle M, McCarten G. The Doppler probe for planning flaps: anatomical study and clinical applications. Br J Plast Surg 1990;43(1):1–16.

31. Kiely J, Kumar M, Wade RG. The accuracy of different modalities of perforator mapping for unilateral DIEP flap breast reconstruction: a systematic review and meta-analysis. J Plast Reconstr Aesthetic Surg 2021;74(5):945–56.

32. Hallock GG. Doppler sonography and color duplex imaging for planning a perforator flap. Clin Plast Surg 2003;30(3):347–57.

33. Imai R, Matsumura H, Tanaka K, et al. Comparison of Doppler sonography and multidetector-row computed tomography in the imaging findings of the deep inferior epigastric perforator artery. Ann Plast Surg 2008;61(1):94–8.

34. Rozen WM, Phillips TJ, Ashton MW, et al. Preoperative imaging for DIEA perforator flaps: a comparative study of computed tomographic angiography and Doppler ultrasound. Plast Reconstr Surg 2008;121(1):9–16.

35. Chen X, Xu Y, Xiao M, et al. Study of distribution of dominant perforators arising from peroneal artery with color Doppler flow imaging and its clinical significance for sural neurocutaneous flap. Zhonghua Zhengxing Waike Zazhi 2010;26(6):417–21.

36. Patel RS, Higgins KM, Enepekides DJ, et al. Clinical utility of colour flow Doppler ultrasonography in planning anterolateral thigh flap harvest. J Otolaryngol Head Neck Surg 2010;39(5).

37. Chim H. Suprafascial radiological characteristics of the superthin profunda artery perforator flap. J Plast Reconstr Aesthetic Surg 2022;75(7):2064–9.

38. Mast BA. Comparison of magnetic resonance angiography and digital subtraction angiography for

visualization of lower extremity arteries. Ann Plast Surg 2001;46(3):261–4.

39. Fukaya E, Grossman RF, Saloner D, et al. Magnetic resonance angiography for free fibula flap transfer. J Reconstr Microsurg 2007;23(04):205–11.

40. Rozen WM, Stella DL, Bowden J, et al. Advances in the pre-operative planning of deep inferior epigastric artery perforator flaps: Magnetic resonance angiography. Microsurgery 2009;29(2):119–23.

41. Schaverien MV, Ludman CN, Neil-Dwyer J, et al. Contrast-enhanced magnetic resonance angiography for preoperative imaging of deep inferior epigastric artery perforator flaps: advantages and disadvantages compared with computed tomography angiography: a United Kingdom perspective. Ann Plast Surg 2011;67(6):671–4.

42. Kruskal JB, Newman PA, Sammons LG, et al. Optimizing Doppler and color flow US: application to hepatic sonography. Radiographics 2004;24(3):657–75.

43. Debelmas A, Camuzard O, Aguilar P, et al. Reliability of color Doppler ultrasound imaging for the assessment of anterolateral thigh flap perforators: a prospective study of 30 perforators. Plast Reconstr Surg 2018;141(3):762–6.

44. Dietrich CF. EFSUMB course book on ultrasound: Lehrbuch und Atlas des endoskopischen Ultraschalls. Latimer Trend Limited. Med Ultrason 2012. https://doi.org/10.11152/mu.2013.2066.153.cfd1lr2.

45. Kehrer A, Sachanadani NS, da Silva NPB, et al. Step-by-step guide to ultrasound-based design of alt flaps by the microsurgeon—basic and advanced applications and device settings. J Plast Reconstr Aesthetic Surg 2020;73(6):1081–90.

46. Sharma M, Hollerbach S, Fusaroli P, et al. General principles of image optimization in EUS. Endosc Ultrasound 2021;10(3):168.

47. Connell MJ, Wu TS. Bedside musculoskeletal ultrasonography. Crit Care Clin 2014;30(2):243–73.

48. Saba L, Atzeni M, Rozen WM, et al. Non-invasive vascular imaging in perforator flap surgery. Acta Radiol 2013;54(1):89–98.

49. Misher JM, Galmer AM, Weinberg MW, et al. Re-evaluating the appropriateness of non-invasive arterial vascular imaging and diagnostic modalities. Curr Treat Options Cardiovasc Med 2017;19:1–22.

50. Kehrer A, Hsu MY, Chen YT, et al. Simplified profunda artery perforator (PAP) flap design using power Doppler ultrasonography (PDU): A prospective study. Microsurgery 2018;38(5):512–23.

51. Haddock NT, Greaney P, Otterburn D, et al. Predicting perforator location on preoperative imaging for the profunda artery perforator flap. Microsurgery 2012;32(7):507–11.

52. Nanno M, Kodera N, Tomori Y, et al. Color Doppler ultrasound assessment for identifying perforator arteries of the second dorsal metacarpal flap. J Orthop Surg 2017;25(1). 2309499016684744.

53. Wang Y, Chang Y, Li S, et al. Methods and effects of high-frequency color Doppler ultrasound assisted reverse island flap of dorsal digital artery of ulnar thumb for repairing skin and soft tissue defects in the distal end of the same finger. Zhonghua Shaoshang Zazhi 2021;37(6):555–61.

54. Pauchot J, Aubry S, Rodiere E, et al. Color doppler ultrasound evaluation of thoracodorsal pedicle quality after axillary lymph node dissection. A way to increase latissimus dorsi flap reliability: about 74 patients. Ann Chir Plast Esthet 2008;112–9.

55. Tashiro K, Yamashita S, Araki J, et al. Preoperative color Doppler ultrasonographic examination in the planning of thoracodorsal artery perforator flap with capillary perforators. J Plast Reconstr Aesthetic Surg 2016;69(3):346–50.

56. Chim H. The Superthin Profunda Artery Perforator Flap for Extremity Reconstruction: Clinical Implications. Plast Reconstr Surg 2022;150(4):915–8.

57. Hong JP, Chung IW. The superficial fascia as a new plane of elevation for anterolateral thigh flaps. Ann Plast Surg 2013;70(2):192–5.

58. Polańska A, Dańczak-Pazdrowska A, Jałowska M, et al. Current applications of high-frequency ultrasonography in dermatology. Postepy Dermatol Alergol 2017;34(6):535–42.

59. Jasaitiene D, Valiukeviciene S, Linkeviciute G, et al. Principles of high-frequency ultrasonography for investigation of skin pathology. J Eur Acad Dermatol Venereol 2011;25(4):375–82.

60. Gong J, Jia Y, Luo W, et al. Preoperative high-frequency color Doppler ultrasound assessment of the blood vessels of the fibular myocutaneous flap. J Plast Reconstr Aesthetic Surg 2022;75(11):3964–9.

61. Xiao H, Shi Y, Wang H, et al. Application of high frequency color Doppler ultrasound in anterolateral thigh flap surgery. Zhongguo Xiu Fu Chong Jian Wai Ke Za Zhi 2013;27(2):178–81.

62. Guo Y, Wei Z, Zeng K, et al. Application of high frequency color Doppler ultrasound combined with wide-field imaging in the preoperative navigation of anterolateral thigh perforator flap surgery. Zhongguo Xiu Fu Chong Jian Wai Ke Za Zhi 2019;33(2):190–4.

63. Visconti G, Bianchi A, Hayashi A, et al. Pure skin perforator flap direct elevation above the subdermal plane using preoperative ultra-high frequency ultrasound planning: a proof of concept. J Plast Reconstr Aesthetic Surg 2019;72(10):1700–38.

64. Visconti G, Hayashi A, Yoshimatsu H, et al. Ultra-high frequency ultrasound in planning capillary perforator flaps: preliminary experience. J Plast Reconstr Aesthetic Surg 2018;71(8):1146–52.

65. Hayashi A, Hayashi N, Yoshimatsu H, et al. Effective and efficient lymphaticovenular anastomosis using preoperative ultrasound detection technique of

lymphatic vessels in lower extremity lymphedema. J Surg Oncol 2018;117(2):290–8.

66. Mihara M, Hara H, Kawakami Y. Ultrasonography for classifying lymphatic sclerosis types and deciding optimal sites for lymphatic-venous anastomosis in patients with lymphoedema. J Plast Reconstr Aesthetic Surg 2018;71(9):1274–81.

67. Kim HB, Jung SS, Cho M-J, et al. Comparative analysis of preoperative high frequency color Doppler ultrasound versus MR lymphangiography versus ICG lymphography of lymphatic vessels in lymphovenous anastomosis. J Reconstr Microsurg 2023; 39(02):92–101.

Superficial Circumflex Iliac Artery Perforator Flap Reconstruction of the Upper Extremity

Caleb W. Barnhill, MD[a], Mark A. Greyson, MD[a,b,c], Matthew L. Iorio, MD[a,b,c],*

KEYWORDS

• SCIP • Extremity reconstruction • Hand • Perforator flap • Microsurgery • Superthin

KEY POINTS

- The superficial circumflex iliac artery perforator (SCIP) flap can be raised as a super thin perforator flap making it an ideal option for soft tissue reconstruction of the hand.
- The primary challenge in harvesting an SCIP flap is related to the variable vascular anatomy of the superficial circumflex iliac artery flap (SCIA) and its associated perforator vessels.
- Major benefits of SCIP flap utilization include minimal donor site morbidity and single-stage reconstruction.
- The SCIP flap can be designed accordingly and reliably as a thin or super thin flap, whereas the classic groin flap requires multiple secondary operations for flap division, debulking, and contouring.
- The angiosomes of the deep and superficial perforator systems have been reliably demonstrated to be inferolateral to the anterior superior iliac spine and along the lateral aspect of the inguinal ligament, respectively.

INTRODUCTION

The attributes and functional characteristics of the upper extremity present a challenge for the reconstruction of soft tissue defects. Reconstruction in the upper extremity includes soft tissue defects secondary to trauma, burns, malignancy, infection, as well as degenerative, congenital, and inflammatory conditions. Whenever possible, reconstruction should seek to restore function and provide a durable reconstruction, while minimizing donor site morbidity.

An emphasis on limb and length preservation has continued to highlight the importance of reconstructive surgery in the management of both upper and lower extremity injuries and wounds. The superficial circumflex iliac artery perforator (SCIP) flap remains a workhorse in the armamentarium of the reconstructive surgeon.

HISTORY

The SCIP, and its predecessor, the superficial circumflex iliac artery flap (SCIA) present unique and powerful options for reconstruction of the upper extremity. Pioneered by McGregor and Jackson in 1972 for the reconstruction of hand defects, the SCIA free flap (sometimes referred to as the "groin flap") was the first successful free fasciocutaneous flap performed.[1] Originally described as a pedicled

ᵃ Division of Plastic and Reconstructive Surgery, University of Colorado Hospital Anschutz Medical Center, Aurora, CO, USA; ᵇ Plastic and Reconstructive Surgery Division of Hand Surgery, University of Colorado Hospital Anschutz Medical Center, Aurora, CO, USA; ᶜ Orthoplastics, Wound and Nerve Surgery, University of Colorado Hospital Anschutz Medical Center, Aurora, CO, USA
* Corresponding author.
E-mail address: matt.iorio@cuanschutz.edu

flap, the reconstructive process required multiple operations including flap division, contouring, and debulking procedures. The average reconstruction required 4.6 surgeries per patient.[2] With the advent of microsurgery and improvement in surgical technique, the SCIP flap has been successfully employed as a free flap for single-stage reconstruction in the upper extremity and hand.

A descendant of the tubed groin flap, there have been advances in both surgical technique and an understanding of flap anatomy, namely, the introduction of perforator flaps which addressed challenges associated with free groin flaps. Koshima introduced the superficial circumflex iliac artery perforator flap nearly 2 decades ago and with it ushered in a new era of extremity reconstruction.[3] The SCIP flap is based on an area with thin adipose tissue in patients with a variety of body habitus and can be elevated in a superthin plane. Superthin, or just "thin," flaps have been implemented as a modification of the original SCIP flap wherein the design of the flap allows for thin pliable tissue reconstruction without the need for secondary flap debulking. Prior outcomes of superthin flaps have also been described by the senior author for design and elevation of both SCIP and anterolateral thigh f flaps for extremity reconstruction.[4,5] Based on this concept, a thin flap is elevated at the superficial fascia, maintaining perforator arborization in the subdermal tissues. This can provide a reliable, well perfused flap. The superthin SCIP has been successfully utilized for head and neck reconstruction and well as defects of the upper extremity. A prospective analysis of 41 superthin SCIP flaps (1.5 mm–4 mm flap thickness) found 98% flap success rate with complete wound healing in 90% of flaps within 3 weeks.[6] Since its inception, there have been various variations including neurotization and inclusion of an osseous and/or muscle component.

ANATOMY

The SCIP flap and its predecessor, the groin flap, are based on the superficial circumflex iliac artery. The origin of the SCIA is typically 3 cm below the inguinal ligament with several variations in vascular branching patterns although the vascular pedicle runs parallel to the inguinal ligament. Generally, the SCIA originates from the femoral artery (70%) or the superficial epigastric artery (30%).[7] The SCIA has a deep (lateral) and superficial (medial) division. The deep branch originates at the medial aspect of the sartorius while the superficial branch is found at the lateral aspect of the sartorius where it pierces the fascia and runs distal to the inguinal ligament and laterally toward the

anterior superior iliac spine (ASIS). Both the superficial and deep branches of the SCIA give off perforators that can be utilized for the SCIP flap. These are termed the "superficial/medial" and "deep/lateral" perforator systems.

The superficial perforator runs laterally and cephalad after piercing the deep fascia and crosses the inguinal ligament at the lateral third. The superficial branch gives off several perforating branches before piercing the superficial fascia and terminating as a major perforating vessel. The deep branch of the SCIA continues in a subfascial course after originating off the SCIA and supplies perfusion to the deep inguinal lymph nodes and the sartorius muscle. At the lateral border of the sartorius, the deep branch pierces both the deep and superficial fascia and gives off several perforating vessels which are concentrated inferior and lateral to the ASIS.

Zubler and colleagues published a study evaluating the anatomic reliability of the SCIP flap and found a clear medio-lateral division. The superficial branch's main perforators gather around the lateral half of the inguinal ligament while the main perforators from the deep branch can be found in a region latero-inferior to the ASIS (**Fig. 1** and **2**).[8] The deep perforator pierces the deep fascia variably whereas the superficial perforator typically perforates the deep fascia 1.5 cm superior and 4.5 cm lateral to the pubic tubercle.

Sinna and colleagues published a study focusing on the reliability and utility of designing the SCIP flap based on a deep branch perforator and found on average that a single dominant perforator originating from the deep branch can

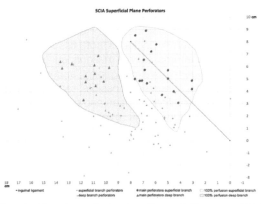

Fig. 1. Mapping of the location of the superficial plane perforators from both the superficial and deep branches of the superficial circumflex iliac artery flap (SCIA).[19] Cédric Zubler et al., The anatomical reliability of the superficial circumflex iliac artery perforator (SCIP) flap, Annals of Anatomy - Anatomischer Anzeiger, 234, 2021, 151624, https://doi.org/10.1016/j.aanat.2020.151624.

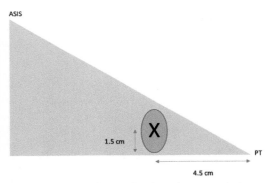

Fig. 2. Location of superficial perforator relative to the pubic tubercle (PT) and anterior superior iliac spine (ASIS).

perfuse skin surface area of 162 cm² with a maximum surface area of 375 cm².[9]

The benefit of a deep branch–based flap is an increase in pedicle length and generally thinner flaps in the absence of debulking. Zubler and team found that on average the superficial branch pedicle length is 6.6 cm ± 1.1 cm while the deep branch pedicle is 9.9 cm ± 1.0 cm. However, most surgeons prefer to utilize a superficial branch perforator due to ease of dissection. Both the perforator artery and concomitant vein are typically less than 1 mm in diameter.

The flap can be neurotized with harvest of the lateral cutaneous branch of the 12th thoracic subcostal nerve. The nerve is located approximately 5 cm posterior to the ASIS, and the nerve can be traced after piercing both the internal and external oblique musculature laterally.[10] The 12th thoracic subcostal nerve should not be confused with the lateral femoral cutaneous nerve (LFCN), which courses below the inguinal ligament and can be located medial to the ASIS and anterior to the sartorius muscle. Injury to the LFCN can result in anterolateral thigh paresthesias.

PRE-OPERATIVE ASSESSMENT

Pre-operative considerations include detailed history and physical examination of both the donor and recipient sites. The nature of the injury should be assessed within the context of the reconstructive plan. Certainly, structural and functional deficits should be considered when choosing the appropriate flap such as prior burns, inguinal hernia/repairs, or stenting and revascularization of the common or superficial femoral arteries. It is paramount to assess for surgical scars or signs of previous trauma at the donor site prior to flap harvest. Additional considerations include viable recipient vessels, zone of injury, and wound contamination.

Patient-related factors including smoking history, diabetes, immunosuppression, radiotherapy, peripheral vascular disease, and obesity need to be considered, and if possible, optimized prior to reconstruction.

The necessity of pre-operative imaging is a source of debate. The vascular anatomy is variable and therefore many surgeons recommend a contrast pre-operative computed tomography (CT) to evaluate the vascular pattern, citing a decrease in harvest time and improvement in flap harvest safety.[11] However, others argue that cross-sectional imaging is superfluous as highlighted by the work of Pereira and colleagues who found that in 100% of cases (N = 43), the pre-operative CT and handheld doppler were concordant regarding the location of the perforator vessels.[12] (**Fig. 3**).

SURGICAL TECHNIQUE

Pre-operative markings include a line from the groin crease to the ASIS, as well as the pubic tubercle to the ASIS. The line along the groin crease and ASIS denotes the orientation of the flap axis. The line between the pubic tubercle and ASIS marks the inguinal ligament, below which the SCIP perforators will be located (**Fig. 4**). Handheld doppler is used to mark the perforators at the skin level in corroboration with the pre-operative CT. The extent of the flap is outlined based upon the

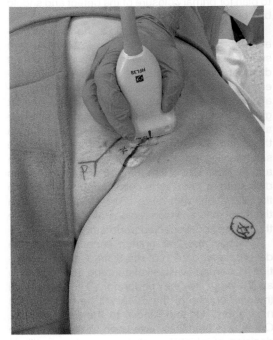

Fig. 3. Evaluation of the deep and superficial superficial circumflex iliac artery perforator (SCIP) perforator using duplex ultrasound.

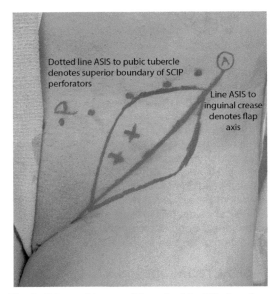

Fig. 4. Skin markings and Doppler-identified perforators for the SCIP flap. The ASIS is denoted by "A," and the line along the inguinal crease denotes the flap axis and elliptical flap design. The pubic tubercle is denoted by "P" and the line A-P denotes the superior boundary of the SCIP perforators at the inguinal crease. Two perforators are denoted by "X."

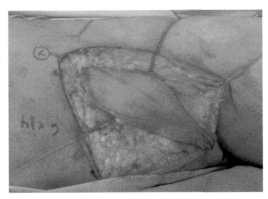

Fig. 5. Flap dissection maintained with lateral tension.

reconstructive requirements of the defect. The width of the flap is typically limited to 8 to 10 cm to plan for primary closure of the defect and should be confirmed with a "pinch test."

Dissection is typically begun along the inferolateral aspect of the flap. The flap is elevated in a suprafascial plane between the superficial and deep fat, which is most easily appreciated inferolaterally. In addition to visualization of the white coloration and fibrous nature of Scarpa's fascia, the fat globules tend to be smaller in the superficial plane and larger deep to this fascial layer. Dissection in this plane is relatively avascular. The authors use self-retaining hook retractors to achieve tension and facilitate dissection (**Figs. 5** and **6**). Hong has described a "hot zone/cold zone" approach to flap elevation, with more rapid elevation through the cold zone or those regions of the flap outside the marked or suspected perforator.[13]

Typically, the first branch encountered is the deep (lateral) branch of the SCIA. Careful dissection is carried while skeletonizing the vessel to avoid injury to the perforator. The superficial (medial) branch of the SCIA will be encountered next and is located medial to the deep branch. Once both branches have been skeletonized, the decision of which branch is isolated and utilized as the flap pedicle should be based upon the specific requirements of the reconstruction and

surgeon preference. The authors typically clamp the deep branch with an Acland clamp and evaluate irrigation of the perforator using intraoperative indocyanine angiography (**Fig. 7**). In most cases, perfusion to the flap based on the superficial branch is robust.

The advantage of the superficial branch is primarily related to the suprafascial course of the vessel and the ease of dissection in isolating the pedicle. In some cases, either due to concerns regarding inadequate perfusion based on the superficial branch or need for longer pedicle, the deep branch will be utilized, and the superficial branch is ligated and divided.

There is typically a superficial vein which courses from the ASIS to the pubic tubercle which is preserved and utilized for venous anastomosis if the venae comitantes are not of sufficient caliber. Often, the venae comitantes of both the deep and superficial branch drain into the superficial vein as separate from the arterial segment. In a study reviewing 210 cases of SCIP flaps, Goh and colleagues found that the superficial vein is present in 88% of the cases.[14] Additionally, preservation of the superficial inferior epigastric vein (SIEV) can

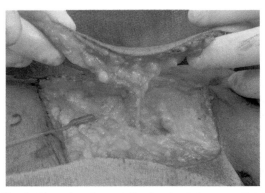

Fig. 6. Flap elevation at the level of the superficial scarpal fascia and dissection of the arterial perforator.

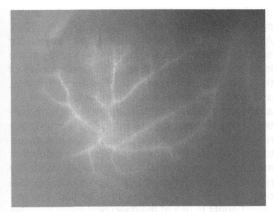

Fig. 7. Indocyanine angiography of SCIP flap and irrigation pattern of superficial (medial) perforator.

be efficacious for additional venous outflow, especially with larger and medially designed flaps. The SIEV typically courses laterally prior to draining into the greater saphenous vein (GSV) near the junction of the femoral vein, while the superficial circumflex iliac vein follows a medial course prior to draining into the GSV. Both venous systems drain the superficial tissues and are paramount for preserving venous outflow following microvascular anastomosis.

SCIP Based on Superficial (Medial) Branch

After ligation and division of the deep branch, the superficial branch is dissected retrograde to its origin. Isolation of the vascular pedicle is carried out through the deep fascia to a length and caliber adequate for successful microsurgical anastomosis. In some cases, the pedicle can be traced retrograde to the SCIA with inclusion of a segment of this vessel in the flap pedicle allowing increased length and vessel caliber.

SCIP Based on the Deep Branch

After ligation and division of the superficial branch, the deep branch is dissected retrograde and is typically noted to pierce the deep and superficial fascia at the lateral aspect of the sartorius muscle. The deep branch provides perfusion to the sartorius muscle and therefore intramuscular dissection is typically required for harvest of the pedicle. Retrograde dissection to the SCIA can be performed to allow increased pedicle length and vessel caliber if required.

FLAP INSET

After appropriate debridement of the upper extremity defect, confirmation of adequate arterial and venous recipient vessels is paramount and should be performed prior to flap division. Typically, microsurgical anastomosis will be performed in an end-to-side fashion for the artery and end-to-end for the vein. The location of the arterial signal should be marked with a suture at the skin level to assist with post-operative monitoring. The appropriate suture for securing the flap must be durable to withstand the dynamic movements of the upper extremity. As such and similar to other procedures involving the glabrous skin, final skin inset is achieved with mattress sutures to maximize wound and dermal eversion. The use of invasive flap monitoring adjuncts such as anastomotic venous flow couplers and doppler blood flow monitors should be at the discretion of the surgeon. However, flap checks with concurrent physical examination are crucial to ensuring flap viability in the early post-operative period, during which most flap failures occur. If utilizing the radial or ulnar arteries for the arterial anastomosis, confirmation of distal perfusion is crucial prior to leaving the operating room.

POST-OPERATIVE MANAGEMENT

The upper extremity should be immobilized for at least 48 to 72 hours to avoid iatrogenic injury to the flap. Frequent monitoring should be implemented into the post-operative care plan with at least 24 hours of hourly flap checks. Post-operative laboratory evaluation should be directed by the patient's clinical course. Post-operative venous thromboembolism prophylaxis regimens vary by institution. Our practice is to administer 81 mg acetylsalicylic acid for 30 days post-operatively with thrice-daily weight-based subcutaneous heparin or enoxaparin while in the hospital. This regimen should be tailored to the patient and any associated coagulopathies or risk factors for deep venous thrombosis /pulmonary embolism. Suture removal should be performed in 2 to 4 weeks depending on wound healing and tension of the closure.

DISCUSSION

The SCIP flap has become a versatile flap in the reconstruction of the upper extremity, and particularly the hand, due to its thin, pliable, and reliable nature (**Figs. 8 and 9**). **Figs. 8 and 9** illustrate the use of an SCIP flap for reconstruction of a finger defect secondary to melanoma resection. Additional benefits of the SCIP flap include ease of harvest and minimal donor site morbidity. The flap is typically harvested in 30 to 60 minutes and the donor site can be closed primarily in most cases.

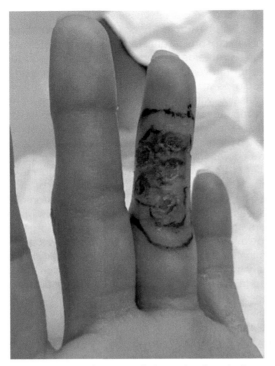

Fig. 8. Large melanoma of the volar fourth finger requiring full thickness resection of soft tissue, digital nerve, and flexor sheath.

The SCIP flap can be customized as a composite flap with inclusion of bone, lymph node, nerve, fascia, and/or subcutaneous fat. The versatility of the SCIP flap provides a robust reconstructive option for head and neck defects as well as extremity reconstruction. There are inherent limitations to

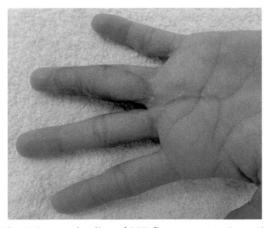

Fig. 9. Post-op healing of SCIP flap reconstruction, utilizing proper digital artery from radial third finger and dorsal vein of third finger. Inset demonstrating return of flexion creases along the thin flap and good range of motion.

the SCIP flap including vessel diameter which can be mitigated with inclusion of the SCIA. Although many studies have mapped perforator anatomy, there remains vascular variability in the location of the perforators and the branching of the SCIA. Pre-operative cross-sectional imaging, and certainly intra-operative handheld doppler examination, provides a roadmap for pedicle dissection. The pedicled and free groin flap remain in the reconstructive repository. However, the disadvantages include need for flap division, contouring, and debulking procedures. There is variability regarding utilization of the deep versus superficial perforators when designing an SCIP flap. The primary benefit to use of the deep perforator includes a longer pedicle at the expense of intramuscular dissection. The choice of perforator branch should be tailored to the reconstructive requirements of the patient as well as surgeon preference. Approximately 90% of SCIP flaps are harvested based on the superficial branch with flap size ranging from 17.5 to 216 cm^2 in a review of 210 SCIP flaps reported by Goh and colleagues[14]

As previously mentioned, various modifications to the SCIP flap have been described. The sartorius can be harvested, in part or whole, as a musculocutaneous SCIP flap. Yang and colleagues evaluated the neurovascular anatomy of the sartorius, finding that the muscle is composed of multiple subunits each with an associated neurovascular hilum. This study highlights the ability to divide the muscle into functional subunits with segmental muscle transfer.[15] In the absence of required muscle bulk, segmental muscle transfer decreases the morbidity associated with harvest of a pelvic stabilizer muscle.

Reconstructive surgeons have incorporated lymph node harvest into SCIP flaps for the treatment of upper extremity lymphedema as well as soft tissue defects. Inguinal lymph nodes (zone 4) can be included within the SCIP harvest as a composite flap and utilized as vascularized lymph node transfer. Osteocutaneous SCIP flaps can be designed to include a portion of the iliac crest for the reconstruction of upper extremity defects. Yoshimatsu and colleagues compared the outcome of SCIA-based iliac bone flaps with traditional fibula flap transfers and found no statistically significant difference in outcomes when comparing pedicle length, rate of bony union or donor, and recipient site complication.[16] The authors found that up to 8 × 3 cm of the iliac crest can successfully be procured and used for reconstruction of small to moderate bony defects.

Utilization of the lateral cutaneous branch of the 12th thoracic subcostal nerve allows for neurotization of the SCIP flap. The option for sensory reconstruction in combination with its thin composition makes the SCIP flap a superb option for reconstruction of the hand and digits. Iida and colleagues published a study outlining the various modifications to the SCIP flap and its clinical applications including thick, super thin, sensate, vascularized bone (iliac crest), supercharged (using intercostal artery perforators [ICAP's]), vascularized groin lymph nodes, and conjoint flap with deep inferior epigastric perforator artery .[17] These variations highlight the utility of the SCIP flap and its many clinical applications, especially in the reconstruction of the upper extremity. Reconstruction of volar digit defects presents a uniquely challenging reconstruction of the upper extremity. Riesel and colleagues described successful SCIP flap reconstruction of a volar thumb burn in a patient exposed to hydrofluoric acid thus highlighting the reconstructive versatility of the SCIP flap.[18]

CLINICAL CASE STUDY

A 33-year-old right hand-dominant male employed as a solar installation electrician sustained a high voltage electrocution with resultant left first webspace wound contracture (**Figs. 10–13**). The patient was initially managed with skin grafting to the left first webspace; however, the graft failed, and the patient developed significant wound

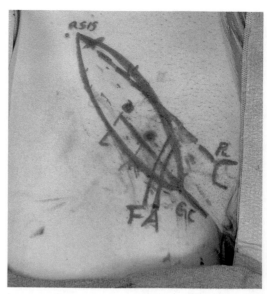

Fig. 11. Right groin SCIP perforator with 10 cm × 5 cm flap designed and centered around the perforator.

contracture with notable functional limitation in the use of his left thumb. On examination, the patient was also noted to have a non-healing wound with tracking to the metacarpophalangeal joint. An Allen's test was performed revealing questionable ulnar artery perfusion to the thumb. The burn wound contracture measured 8 × 4 cm. The patient was noted to be without trauma to the groin region. The reconstructive options were reviewed with the patient and ultimately a superficial circumflex iliac perforator flap was chosen for reconstruction of the left first webspace burn wound contracture. A pre-operative left upper extremity angiogram was obtained which notably revealed absence of the left ulnar artery at the wrist.

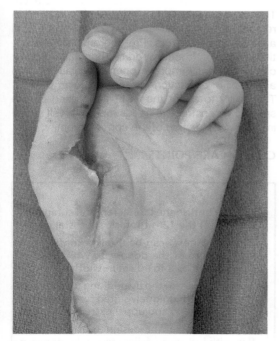

Fig. 10. Pre-operative left first webspace burn contracture, with unstable scar tissue and thumb adduction.

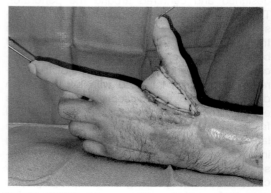

Fig. 12. SCIP flap inset to first webspace with thin, pliable tissue.

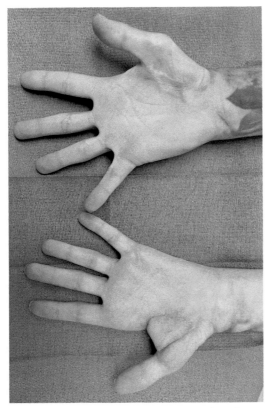

Fig. 13. Healing flap with correction of adduction contracture and improved thumb and webspace range of motion at 6 weeks postoperatively.

OPERATIVE TECHNIQUE

A regional block of the left upper extremity was performed prior to the patient entering to operative suite. After induction of general anesthesia, a tourniquet was applied to the left upper extremity. Handheld doppler was used to localize the right groin SCIP perforator with a 10 × 5 cm flap designed and centered around the perforator. The authors began by excising the left first webspace burn scar contracture to the level of the thenar fascia. The recipient vessels were isolated based on the pre-operative angiogram (dorsal subcutaneous vein and radial artery). The SCIP perforators were again localized with intra-operative doppler prior to flap dissection. The flap was elevated from lateral to medial along the superficial fascia with identification and preservation of the lateral and deep perforators. A large vein draining into the femoral system was isolated and preserved. The medial system was provisionally clamped and indocyanine green (ICG) angiography was performed to ensure adequate perfusion based on the lateral system. Once confirmed, the medial vascular system was divided. The lateral perforator was isolated to the takeoff from the femoral artery through the fascia of the sartorius muscle. Utilizing intra-operative microscope, the microvascular anastomosis was completed using a 2.5 mm venous coupler (SCIP vein to superficial dorsal vein) and a hand sewn end-to-side arterial anastomosis of the lateral SCIP perforator to the radial artery. The site of cutaneous arterial doppler signal was marked with a Prolene suture and the flap was inset with 4 to 0 Nylon mattress sutures. A Vioptix probe was placed for post-operative flap monitoring.

SUMMARY

Originally viewed as a suitable option for reconstruction of the upper extremity, the pedicled and free groin flap became a workhorse primarily due to minimal donor site morbidity. Unfortunately, flap debulking and contouring procedures in addition to flap division required multiple subsequent operations to complete the reconstruction. With the advent of the perforator flap and advances in microsurgery, the SCIP flap has become an excellent option for reconstruction in the upper extremity due to capacity to elevate in a superthin plane and ability to harvest as a chimeric flap. Challenges to utilization of the SCIP flap include small vessel diameter and a short pedicle length, primarily when basing the flap on the superficial branch. The largest variable in designing the SCIP flap remains the vascular anatomy of the SCIA and associated perforators. Pre-operative CT evaluation in addition to intra-operative handheld doppler can significantly improve operative planning and assist with dissection of the vascular pedicle. The ability to adapt the SCIP flap based on the specific reconstructive needs makes it well suited in the reconstruction of the upper extremity.

CLINICS CARE POINTS

- Do not confuse the lateral femoral cutaneous nerve with the 12th thoracic subcostal nerve.
- The "pinch test" can be used to confirm primary closure of the donor site which is typically limited to 8 to 10 cm in width.
- The thin nature of the tissue along the inguinal crease makes it uniquely suited for reconstruction of the hand and upper extremity.
- The SCIP flap can be designed as a chimeric flap with inclusion of iliac crest, subcutaneous fat, inguinal lymph nodes, 12 thoracic subcostal nerve, and fascia.

- The majority of SCIP flaps can be harvested based on the superficial (medial) branch perforator with a portion of the SCIA included in the pedicle if added length or vessel caliber is required.
- Harvest of the SCIP flap based on the deep (lateral) branch perforator provides a longer pedicle but requires intramuscular dissection of the sartorius.
- Adequate perfusion of the flap can be confirmed with intra-operative indocyanine angiography prior to ligation of the secondary perforator.
- The superficial branch's main perforators gather around the lateral half of the inguinal ligament while the main perforators from the deep branch can be found in a region latero-inferior to the ASIS.

DISCLOSURE

The authors have no financial interests in any of the products or techniques mentioned and have received no external support related to this study.

REFERENCES

1. McGregor IA, Jackson IT. The groin flap. Br J Plast Surg 1972;25:3–16.
2. Goertz O, Kapalschinski N, Daigeler A, et al. The effectiveness of pedicled groin flaps in the treatment of hand defects: results of 49 patients. J Hand Surg Am 2012;37(10):2088–94.
3. Koshima I, Nanba Y, Tsutsui T, et al. Superficial circumflex iliac artery perforator flap for reconstruction of limb defects. Plast Reconstr Surg 2004;113(1):233–40.
4. Diamond S, Seth AK, Chattha AS, et al. Outcomes of Subfascial, Suprafascial, and Super-Thin Anterolateral Thigh Flaps. Tailoring Thickness without Added Morbidity 2017;34(03):176–84.
5. Seth AK, Iorio ML. Super-Thin and Suprafascial Anterolateral Thigh Perforator Flaps for Extremity Reconstruction 2017;33(07):466–73.
6. Lee KT, Park B, Kim Eun Kyung, et al. Superthin SCIP Flap for Reconstruction of Subungual Melanoma 2017;140(6):1278–89.
7. Chung KC. Operative techniques in plastic surgery. Wolters Kluwer; 2020. p. 5108.
8. Zubler C, Haberthür D, Hlushchuk R, et al. The anatomical reliability of the superficial circumflex iliac artery perforator (SCIP) flap. Annals of Anatomy - Anatomischer Anzeiger. 2021;234:151624.
9. Sinna R, Hajji H, Qassemyar Q, et al. Anatomical background of the perforator flap based on the deep branch of the superficial circumflex iliac artery (SCIP Flap): a cadaveric study. Eplasty 2010;10:e11.
10. Chung KC. Operative techniques in plastic surgery. Wolters Kluwer; 2020. p. 5111.
11. He Y, Jin S, Tian Z, et al. Superficial circumflex iliac artery perforator flap's imaging, anatomy and clinical applications in oral maxillofacial reconstruction 2016;44(3):242–8.
12. Pereira N, Parada L, Kufeke M, et al. A New Planning Method to Easily Harvest the Superficial Circumflex Iliac Artery Perforator Flap. J Reconstr Microsurg 2019;36(03):165–70.
13. Kehrer A, Sachanadani NS, Silva, et al. Step-by-step guide to ultrasound-based design of alt flaps by the microsurgeon – Basic and advanced applications and device settings. J Plast Reconstr Aesthetic Surg 2020;73(6):1081–90.
14. Goh TLH, Park SW, Cho JY, et al. The Search for the Ideal Thin Skin Flap. Plast Reconstr Surg 2015;135(2):592–601.
15. Yang D, Morris SF, Sigurdson L. The sartorius muscle: anatomic considerations for reconstructive surgeons. Surg Radiol Anat 1998;20(5):307–10.
16. Yoshimatsu H, Iida T, Yamamoto T, et al. Superficial Circumflex Iliac Artery-Based Iliac Bone Flap Transfer for Reconstruction of Bony Defects. J Reconstr Microsurg 2018;34(9):719–28.
17. Iida T. Superficial Circumflex Iliac Perforator (SCIP) Flap: Variations of the SCIP Flap and Their Clinical Applications. J Reconstr Microsurg 2014;30(07):505–8.
18. Riesel J, Giladi A, Iorio M. Volar Resurfacing of the Thumb with a Superficial Circumflex Iliac Artery Perforator Flap after Hydrofluoric Acid Burn. Journal of Hand and Microsurgery 2018;10(03):162–5.
19. Els-cdn.com. Published 2023. Available at: https://ars.els-cdn.com/content/image/1-s2.0-S0940960220301680-gr4_lrg.jpg. Accessed May 23, 2023

Thin Profunda Artery Perforator Flap for Hand and Upper Extremity Coverage

Isaac Smith, BA, Ramin Shekouhi, MD, Markos Mardourian, BS, Harvey Chim, MD*

KEYWORDS

- Hand • Upper extremity • Free flap • Profunda artery perforator flap, • PAP flap • Thin PAP flap
- Soft tissue coverage

KEY POINTS

- In the hand and upper extremity, thin flaps are preferred for a reconstruction with comparable thickness to the natural tissue.
- The thin profunda artery perforator flap is a reliable flap option with a large perforasome supporting a large skin paddle for defect contouring.
- Preoperative CT angiography or color Doppler ultrasonography can map the dominant perforator and assist in harvesting thin or superthin flaps efficiently and safely.

INTRODUCTION

The profunda artery perforator (PAP) flap has recently gained popularity for use in free tissue transfer. For reconstruction in the breast or head and neck, it provides a sizable thickness and bulk of vascularized tissue, with the advantages of a concealed donor site in the posterior medial thigh.[1] The attractiveness of the PAP flap includes the pliability of the skin and subcutaneous fat, reliable anatomic landmarks, sufficient pedicle length, and a hidden donor site.[2] PAP donor sites avoid potential problems found with anterolateral thigh (ALT) flap and transverse myocutaneous gracilis (TMG) flaps. ALT flaps result in a visible scar as well as the occurrence of paresthesia in the distribution of the lateral femoral cutaneous nerve. There is also a risk of lymphatic injury with TMG flaps.[3,4]

Ample soft tissue in the posteromedial thigh and consistent vascular anatomy with "A", "B," and "C "perforators at different locations in the thigh enable PAP flaps to be harvested from different locations and in different configurations to cover a range of defects.[5] The amount and quality of the adipose tissue is suited to breast reconstruction, particularly when limited abdominal tissue is available.[6] However, for areas with thinner skin, such as the extremities, an issue with the PAP flap is the excess tissue that makes for a thicker flap with suboptimal esthetic and functional sequelae.

The thin PAP flap aims to overcome excessive flap thickness through primary thinning, by elevating the flap superficial to Scarpa fascia to achieve a "thin" flap, or in the subcutaneous fat, for a "superthin" flap.[7] Primary thinning of the flap yields a better "like-for-like" reconstruction, achieving a suitable match for reconstruction in the upper and lower extremities.[8,9] In the upper extremities, thin flaps also alleviate the need for intraoperative flap thinning or secondary procedures for debulking.[10] The objective of this review is to provide a comprehensive overview of the existing literature regarding the evolution of PAP flaps in general as well as thin fasciocutaneous

Division of Plastic and Reconstructive Surgery, University of Florida College of Medicine, Gainesville, FL, USA
* Corresponding author. 1600 S.W. Archer Road, Gainesville, FL 32610.
E-mail address: harveychim@yahoo.com

Hand Clin 40 (2024) 189–198
https://doi.org/10.1016/j.hcl.2023.10.002

flaps while discussing use of the thin and superthin PAP flap at our institution for reconstruction in the upper extremity.

HISTORY AND DEVELOPMENT OF PROFUNDA ARTERY PERFORATOR FLAPS

Before the formal description of the "PAP" flap for breast reconstruction in 2012,[2] several authors described flaps based on posterior thigh perforators. Hurteau and colleagues[11] described a posterior thigh V-Y advancement flap based on perforators from the inferior gluteal artery for reconstruction of ischial pressure ulcers. Song and colleagues[12] built an anatomic foundation for thigh-based flaps, highlighting the reliability of perforators in this region. Angrigiani and colleagues, through anatomic dissections, described the anatomy relating to PAPs, describing the "adductor" flap, perfused by cutaneous perforating branches of the profunda femoris artery.[13] This adductor flap has since evolved into what is now known as the PAP flap.

The PAP flap gained traction, particularly for breast reconstruction after Allen and colleagues[2] reported their successful results in 2012. They observed that PAP flaps are a highly favorable option for breast reconstruction due to a long pedicle with the option to anastomose either to internal mammary or thoracodorsal vessels.[2,14] In addition, medial thigh tissue was more malleable for breast reconstruction than abdominal or gluteal donor sites, and patients often preferred esthetic outcomes related to a posterior medial thigh donor site.[2,14] Perforasome analysis of PAP flaps by Wong and colleagues[6] provided much needed information regarding the horizontal and vertical dimensions of PAPs using CT angiography.

Over time, the utilization of PAP flaps has extended beyond breast reconstruction and expanded to encompass the reconstruction of defects in other regions. For head and neck reconstruction, some groups prefer the PAP flap due to its consistent anatomy and better donor site.[3,15,16] A comparative study evaluating the outcomes of PAP flap with ALT flaps for head and neck reconstruction showed equivalent outcomes, with PAP flaps having more perforators with better donor site esthetic outcomes compared with ALT flaps.[15] In addition, though the ALT flap can have variable anatomy[17] complicating flap harvest, the PAP flap has consistent anatomy with a straightforward harvest. The PAP flap has shown favorable results for isolated vulvar reconstruction due to the presence of thin pliable skin and consistent perforator anatomy.[18,19]

For lower extremity reconstruction, the radial forearm (RF), superficial circumflex iliac artery perforator (SCIP), and ALT flaps have been more frequently used compared with PAP flaps.[3,8,20] Nevertheless, there has been a recent increase in the utilization of PAP flaps for extremity reconstruction, primarily using a vertical skin paddle design. Large flaps measuring up to 30 cm in length could be used due to the reliable perfusion of the PAP flap.[21] Although SCIP and RFF flaps are similarly thin and pliable, they can be more challenging to harvest or have an unfavorable donor site.

Good outcomes have been described with the PAP flap for extremity reconstruction.[9,21,22] However, one of the challenges with traditional subfascial PAP flaps, particularly in the upper extremity, is the bulk and thickness of the flap that cannot optimally restore the natural contour of the extremities due to the tapered conical form of the flap. In addition, because defects in the extremities are typically superficial, using a thick flap for reconstruction can lead to unsatisfactory esthetic outcomes and limited functionality. Consequently, this has led to the development of thin and superthin flaps as an alternative approach.

EVOLUTION OF THIN AND SUPERTHIN FLAPS

Early reports of "super-thin" flap design and use by Chinese surgeons described a random pattern pedicle flap based on the subdermal plexus that had been in use since the 1980s.[23,24] Hyakusoku and colleagues designed "super-thin" narrow pedicled occipitocervical and intercostal perforator flaps for use in head and neck reconstruction in 1994.[25] These flaps were thinned secondarily to the level of the subdermal vascular network in the distal half to two-thirds, following initial elevation at the thickness of a conventional skin flap.[25] There were four reasons postulated by Hyakusoku[25] for survival of thinned skin flaps: (1) perfusion through the subdermal vascular plexus; (2) increasing the survival length of the flap by decreasing metabolic load in the distal area of the flap; (3) survival of the distal thinned area of the flap as a free skin graft; and (4) survival of the distal thinned area as both a flap through the subdermal plexus and a graft through plasmatic imbibition.

More recent reports have focused on the elevation of thin superficial SCIP flaps primarily at the junction of the superficial and deep fat.[26,27] Hong and colleagues[27] investigated the outcomes of ALT, SCIP, and gluteal artery perforator flaps elevated on the level of the superficial fascia. Advantages reported with this technique include obviating the need for additional debulking after initial flap elevation and a better contour match in areas with thinner skin. In this series, a flap survival rate of 97% was reported with the largest flap measuring 30 × 18 cm based on a single perforator. Specific to the SCIP flap, primary elevation of thin flaps avoids potential complications associated with extended tissue dissection, such as the risk of lymph node injuries that could occur when dissecting beneath the fascia.[27,28]

Subsequently, the free "pure skin perforator" SCIP flap was described by Narushima and colleagues, elevated deep to the subdermal plexus, with applications in reconstruction of microtia or finger defects.[7,29] Primary elevation of thin flaps resolves challenges associated with secondary flap defatting. Debulking after initial flap elevation can, on occasion, increase the risk of partial flap loss.[30] Microdissection of the pedicle is another option allowing intraoperative flap thinning, although this is time-consuming.[31]

A newer option explored by our group for extremity reconstruction is the thin and superthin PAP flap.[10,32,33] In our series, flaps were elevated either at the level of the superficial fascia or subcutaneous fat with a mean thickness of 0.7 cm, for a "like-for-like" reconstruction in the hand and upper extremity.[10,33] Preoperative localization of the dominant perforator through imaging is essential for this flap.

ANATOMIC LANDMARKS FOR PAP FLAP HARVEST

The profunda femoris artery is the primary blood supply for the thigh. Originating from the postero-lateral side of the femoral artery below the inguinal ligament, the profunda femoris artery gives off medial branches to the adductor compartment, as well as three perforating branches through the adductor magnus muscle to the posterior and medial compartments of the thigh.[34]

The longitudinal axis in the posterior medial thigh where PAPs can be found has been variably described as extending from the pubic tubercle to the medial femoral condyle or from the ischial tuberosity to the semitendinosus tendon insertion. Other authors have used a line posterior and parallel to the gracilis muscle as the axis for locating PAPs.[34–36] In anatomic studies, the origin of the primary perforator was found 7 to 10 cm (mean ≈ 8 cm) distal to the inferior gluteal sulcus.[35–37]

The diameter of the PAP can vary based on the extent of proximal dissection on the pedicle, with an average diameter ranging from 0.8 to 2.5 mm.[34–36] The published mean length of the perforator's pedicle from its origin also varies, ranging from 6.8 to 11 cm.[35–39] To achieve an acceptable pedicle length, the perforator should be dissected to its origin.

PREOPERATIVE CONSIDERATIONS FOR ELEVATION OF A THIN OR SUPERTHIN PROFUNDA ARTERY PERFORATOR FLAP

For primary elevation of thin and superthin PAP flaps, the flap is ideally perfused through the dominant or largest perforator in the posterior medial thigh to ensure that the largest perforasome is captured and to reduce risk of partial flap necrosis. Owing to considerable anatomic variation in the location and caliber of PAPs, localizing the dominant perforator can be challenging. Therefore, preoperative imaging is essential for flap planning. Although the hand-held Doppler probe is the most common method used for preoperative localization of perforators, it can be associated with high rates of false-positive results.[40,41] In addition, the hand-held Doppler cannot determine the anatomic course or morphology of perforators. Information on the suprafascial course of the perforator is very useful when elevating a suprafascial or thinner PAP flap.

Our approach is to use a combination of computed tomography angiography (CTA) and color Doppler ultrasound (CDU) for localizing and mapping the dominant perforator before design of a thin or superthin PAP flap. Haddock and colleagues[38] reported that CTA was a reliable imaging modality for PAP flap planning with a sensitivity rate of 98.8% for perforator detection.[38] Wong and colleagues[6] confirmed the utility of CTA as an option for accurate PAP mapping.

For thin PAP flaps, the coronal view on CTA allows localization of the approximate proximal-distal (P-D) distance of the dominant perforator along the longitudinal axis in the posterior medial thigh in relation to the groin crease (**Fig. 1**). In this example, the largest perforators on axial cuts were first localized on each thigh and then the P-D distance from the groin crease to each perforator measured on the coronal cut (see **Fig. 1**B). The left-sided PAP was larger (see **Fig. 1**A) and selected as the perforator to design the flap on. Further measurements (see **Fig. 1**C) are then performed to evaluate the distance from the deep fascia to the skin and the distance from the bifurcation point of the perforator to the skin, which provides a guide to the safe thickness of the flap that can be elevated close to the perforator.[10,32] Others[42] have also demonstrated the utility of CTA for preoperative planning of thin PAP flaps for tongue reconstruction. In our series, the mean difference between the preoperative P-D distance of the dominant perforator measured on CTA and the actual intraoperative P-D distance was 1.2 ± 0.6 cm, which was clinically insignificant.[10]

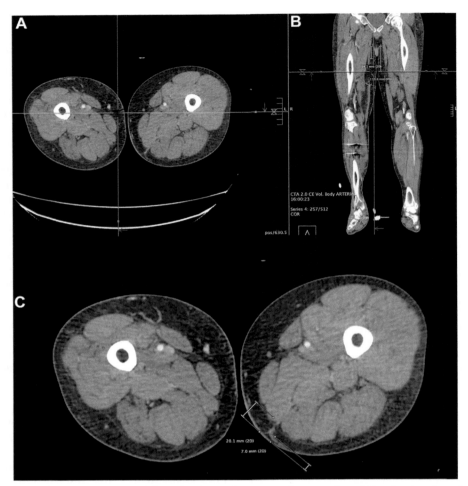

Fig. 1. Example of CTA and CDU used for selection and preoperative mapping of the dominant perforator. (*A*) The largest perforator is found on the left thigh (axial cut). (*B*) Coronal cut is used to measure the distance of the dominant perforator on each thigh from the groin crease. (*C*) Further measurements on axial cut are made of the distance from the deep fascia to the skin (20.1 mm) and the distance from the bifurcation point of the perforator to the skin (7.0 mm). In this case, safe flap elevation in the thin plane close to the perforator would be slightly deeper than 7.0 mm.

CDU is then used immediately before surgery to confirm the location and map the anatomic course of the dominant perforator.[33] In this fashion, CTA is used to grossly locate the PAP to be used preoperatively, followed by finer measurement and assessment of suprafascial anatomy of the perforator on the operating table through CDU.[32]

INTRAOPERATIVE CONSIDERATIONS FOR THIN PROFUNDA ARTERY PERFORATOR FLAP HARVEST

We prefer to harvest the flap from a supine frog leg position. However, others prefer a lithotomy

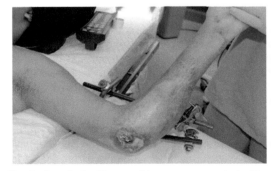

Fig. 2. Case 1: An 18-year-old woman presented with a left medial elbow defect with an exposed plate. Local and pedicled flaps were not possible due to previous surgery in the left arm and forearm. She had concomitant fractures of the left distal humerus and radial head.

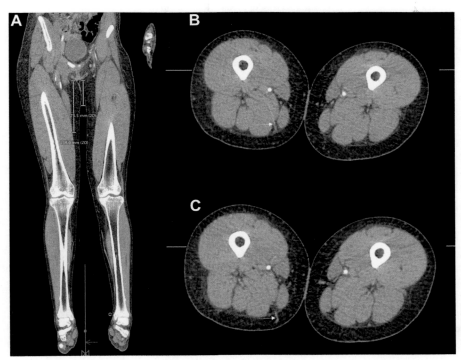

Fig. 3. Case 1: Preoperative CTA used for localization and mapping of the dominant perforator on the right thigh. (*A*) Largest perforator localized on coronal cut 15.5 cm from the groin crease. The dominant perforator (*white arrow*) is visualized in its subfascial (*B*) and suprafascial (*C*) course.

position or "semi-flamingo" position, which is also possible. The flap is centered on the dominant perforator. The anterior incision is made first. Unlike for traditional subfascial flap harvest, dissection proceeds in the subcutaneous plane by beveling inward to reduce the thickness of the flap, until the desired flap thickness is achieved. Further anterior-to-posterior dissection proceeds in the suprascarpal plane for a "thin" flap or the subcutaneous plane for a "superthin" flap until the vicinity of the perforator, posterior to the

gracilis muscle. Then, the fascia is opened in a limited fashion around the perforator and proximal dissection carried on the perforator until sufficient pedicle length and caliber of vessels is achieved. Then, dissection proceeds in the subfascial plane proximal, distal, and posterior to the perforator, to capture a small segment of fascia around the perforator. After this is done, the posterior incision is made, and the flap completely islanded. The rest of the flap is elevated at the desired thickness in the "thin" or "superthin" plane until close to the

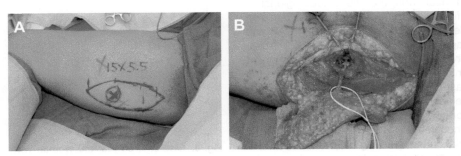

Fig. 4. Case 1: (*A*) A 14 × 5.5 cm superthin PAP flap was designed centered over the dominant perforator on the right thigh. (*B*) Following elevation of the flap.

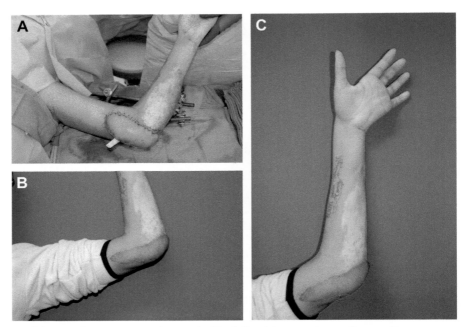

Fig. 5. Case 1: (*A*) Immediate postoperative result. (*B, C*) Short-term postoperative result.

dominant perforator, where careful dissection is carried to connect to the previously dissected suprafascial plane close to the perforator. With the flap completely free, further dissection can be carried proximally on the pedicle if needed to achieve more length.[10,32,33]

CASE EXAMPLES IN UPPER EXTREMITY RECONSTRUCTION
Case 1: Superthin Flap for Medial Elbow Coverage

An 18-year-old woman was referred for flap coverage of wound breakdown and plate exposure at the left medial elbow (**Fig. 2**) after she sustained severe soft tissue injuries following a motor vehicle accident. Owing to prior surgeries and scarring related to a previous anterior interosseous nerve to ulnar deep motor branch nerve transfer and failed local flaps, the use of locoregional or pedicled flaps was not possible. Hence, decision was made to perform a free superthin PAP flap for coverage.

Preoperative CTA showed a larger dominant perforator on the right thigh, 15.5 cm from the groin crease on coronal view (**Fig. 3**A). Axial images were used to follow the course of the dominant perforator in the right thigh from its origin on the profunda femoris artery (see **Fig. 3**B) to its suprafascial course (see **Fig. 3**C). CDU was used before surgery to further localize and map the dominant perforator. In this case, the size of the

skin paddle (14 × 5.5 cm) (**Fig. 4**A) was relatively small. Hence, preoperative imaging was essential for rapid and safe elevation of a superthin flap (see **Fig. 4**B). A shorter pedicle length (6.5 cm) was selected in this case, with the recipient artery being the superior ulnar collateral artery in an end-to-side fashion. **Fig. 5**A–C shows immediate and short-term postoperative results.

Case 2: Thin Flap for Resurfacing of First Webspace Contracture

A 64-year-old woman sustained a full-thickness scald burn resulting in scarring primarily over the dorsoradial aspect of the right hand. She was initially treated with xenograft followed by split-

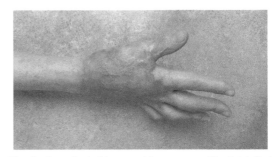

Fig. 6. Case 2: A 64-year-old woman with right first webspace contracture following scald burn to the right hand resurfaced with split thickness skin graft.

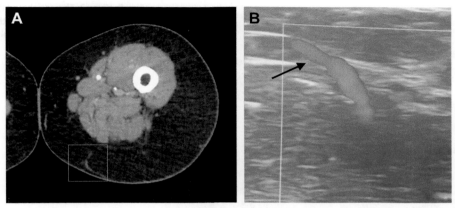

Fig. 7. Case 2: (*A*) Preoperative CTA used for localization of the dominant perforator on the left thigh (white box), showing a "T" suprafascial branching pattern. (*B*) CDU used for further localization and mapping of the dominant perforator. One limb of the suprafascial branching (*arrow*) can be seen on this image.

thickness skin grafts, resulting in secondary scar contracture which resulted in the primary problem of a contracted first webspace (**Fig. 6**). She was unable to oppose or abduct her thumb and could not use her right hand to hold any objects. She was planned for release of the first webspace contracture followed by resurfacing with a thin PAP flap.

Preoperative CTA (**Fig. 7**A) showed a dominant "T" pattern perforator in the right posterior medial thigh 7 cm distal to the groin crease. CDU (see

Fig. 7B) was used to localize and map the perforator before flap elevation. Here, one limb of the suprafascial branching pattern can be seen. A 12 × 5.5 cm skin paddle was designed and elevated in the "thin" plane (**Fig. 8**A). Arterial anastomosis was to the dorsal radial artery. Immediate (see **Fig. 8**B) and 3-month postoperative results are shown (see **Fig. 8**C, D). The concealed donor site on the left thigh cannot be seen from in front (**Fig. 9**A) and is only seen from a posteromedial view (see **Fig. 9**B).

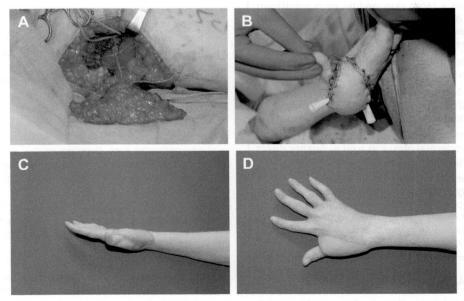

Fig. 8. Case 2: (*A*) A 12 × 5.5 cm flap was elevated on the thin plane. (*B*) Immediate postoperative result. (*C, D*) Three-month postoperative result.

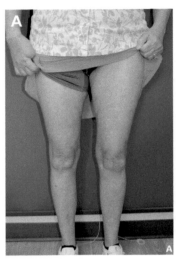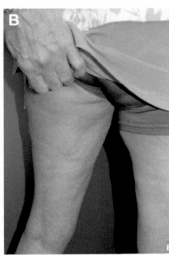

Fig. 9. Case 2: The concealed flap donor site scar cannot be seen from the frontal view (*A*) and can only be visualized from a posteromedial view (*B*).

SUMMARY

The PAP flap, when harvested in the suprafascial, thin or superthin plane, provides a good source of thin pliable tissue for resurfacing of defects in the hand and upper extremity, with a concealed donor site. Preoperative flap planning using CTA or CDU is essential for obtaining information regarding the location and course of the dominant perforator.

CLINICS CARE POINTS

- Profunda artery perforator (PAP) flaps can provide a large skin paddle with significant bulk of subcutaneous tissue that is suited for reconstruction in the breast and head and neck reconstruction.
- Thinner flaps are preferred for extremity reconstruction.
- Thin and superthin PAP flaps can be harvested through flap elevation superficial to Scarpa's fascia or in the subcutaneous fat.
- Thin and superthin PAP flaps are perfused by the subdermal plexus as well as further direct linking vessels in the subcutaneous fat.
- Preoperative flap planning using computed tomography angiography and color Doppler ultrasound is an essential step for identifying the dominant perforator and understanding the underlying vascular anatomy for thin and superthin PAP flaps.

DISCLOSURE

The authors have nothing to disclose. None of the authors have a financial interest in the discussed manuscript. No funding was received for this article.

REFERENCES

1. Allen RJ Jr, Lee Z-H, Mayo JL, et al. The profunda artery perforator flap experience for breast reconstruction. Plast Reconstr Surg 2016;138(5):968–75.
2. Allen RJ, Haddock NT, Ahn CY, et al. Breast reconstruction with the profunda artery perforator flap. Plast Reconstr Surg 2012;129(1):16e–23e.
3. Mayo JL, Canizares O, Torabi R, et al. Expanding the applications of the profunda artery perforator flap. Plast Reconstr Surg 2016;137(2):663–9.
4. Zaussinger M, Tinhofer IE, Hamscha U, et al. A head-to-head comparison of the vascular basis of the transverse myocutaneous gracilis, profunda artery perforator, and fasciocutaneous infragluteal flaps: an anatomical study. Plast Reconstr Surg 2019;143(2):381–90.
5. Largo RD, Chu CK, Chang EI, et al. Perforator mapping of the profunda artery perforator flap: Anatomy and clinical experience. Plast Reconstr Surg 2020; 146(5):1135–45.
6. Wong C, Nagarkar P, Teotia S, et al. The profunda artery perforator flap: investigating the perforasome using three-dimensional computed tomographic angiography. Plast Reconstr Surg 2015;136(5): 915–9.
7. Narushima M, Yamasoba T, Iida T, et al. Pure skin perforator flaps: the anatomical vascularity of the superthin flap. Plast Reconstr Surg 2018;142(3): 351e–60e.
8. Ciudad P, Huang TCT, Manrique OJ, et al. Expanding the applications of the combined transverse upper gracilis and profunda artery perforator (TUGPAP) flap for extensive defects. Microsurgery 2019;39(4):316–25.

9. Boriani F, Sassu P, Atzeni M, et al. The profunda artery perforator flap for upper limb reconstruction: A case report and literature review on the flap applications in reconstruction. Microsurgery 2022;42(7): 714–21.

10. Chim H. The Superthin Profunda Artery Perforator Flap for Extremity Reconstruction: Clinical Implications. Plast Reconstr Surg 2022;150(4):915–8.

11. Hurteau J, Bostwick J, Nahai F, et al. VY advancement of hamstring musculocutaneous flap for coverage of ischial pressure sores. Plast Reconstr Surg 1981;68(4):539–42.

12. Song YG, Chen GZ, Song YL. The free thigh flap: a new free flap concept based on the septocutaneous artery. Br J Plast Surg 1984;37(2):149–59.

13. Angrigiani C, Grilli D, Thorne CH. The adductor flap: a new method for transferring posterior and medial thigh skin. Plast Reconstr Surg 2001;107(7): 1725–31.

14. Blechman KM, Broer PN, Tanna N, et al. Stacked profunda artery perforator flaps for unilateral breast reconstruction: A case report. J Reconstr Microsurg 2013;29(09):631–4.

15. Wu JC, Huang JJ, Tsao CK, et al. Comparison of posteromedial thigh profunda artery perforator flap and anterolateral thigh perforator flap for head and neck reconstruction. Plast Reconstr Surg 2016; 137(1):257–66.

16. Scaglioni MF, Kuo YR, Yang JC, et al. The posteromedial thigh flap for head and neck reconstruction: anatomical basis, surgical technique, and clinical applications. Plast Reconstr Surg 2015;136(2): 363–75.

17. Lakhiani C, Lee MR, Saint-Cyr M. Vascular anatomy of the anterolateral thigh flap: a systematic review. Plast Reconstr Surg 2012;130(6):1254–68.

18. Huang JJ, Chang NJ, Chou HH, et al. Pedicle perforator flaps for vulvar reconstruction—New generation of less invasive vulvar reconstruction with favorable results. Gynecol Oncol 2015;137(1): 66–72.

19. Chang TNJ, Lee CH, Lai CH, et al. Profunda artery perforator flap for isolated vulvar defect reconstruction after oncological resection. J Surg Oncol 2016; 113(7):828–34.

20. Sakai S, Shibata M. Free adductor perforator flap in lower leg reconstruction. J Plast Reconstr Aesthetic Surg 2006;59(9):990–3.

21. Scaglioni MF, Hsieh CH, Giovanoli P, et al. The posteromedial thigh (PMT) flap for lower extremity reconstruction. Microsurgery 2017;37(8):865–72.

22. Ciudad P, Kaciulyte J, Torto FL, et al. The profunda artery perforator free flap for lower extremity reconstruction. Microsurgery 2022;42(1):13–21.

23. Situ P. Pedicled flap with subdermal vascular network. Academic J First Medical College of PLA(Chinese). 1986;6:60.

24. Wang YJ. Clinical application of early division of the pedicle of super-thin skin flap with a subdermal vascular network. Pract J Aesth Plast Surg (Chinese) 1990;1:23–4.

25. Hyakusoku H, Gao JH. The "super-thin" flap. Br J Plast Surg 1994;47(7):457–64.

26. Koshima I, Nanba Y, Tsutsui T, et al. Superficial circumflex iliac artery perforator flap for reconstruction of limb defects. Plast Reconstr Surg 2004; 113(1):233–40.

27. Hong JP, Choi DH, Suh H, et al. A new plane of elevation: the superficial fascial plane for perforator flap elevation. J Reconstr Microsurg 2014;30(07): 491–6.

28. Hong JP, Sun SH, Ben-Nakhi M. Modified superficial circumflex iliac artery perforator flap and supermicrosurgery technique for lower extremity reconstruction: a new approach for moderate-sized defects. Ann Plast Surg 2013;71(4):380–3.

29. Narushima M, Yamasoba T, Iida T, et al. Pure skin perforator flap for microtia and congenital aural atresia using supermicrosurgical techniques. J Plast Reconstr Aesthetic Surg 2011;64(12): 1580–4.

30. Kimura N, Satoh K. Consideration of a thin flap as an entity and clinical applications of the thin anterolateral thigh flap. Plast Reconstr Surg 1996;97(5): 985–92.

31. Kimura N, Saitoh M, Hasumi T, et al. Clinical application and refinement of the microdissected thin groin flap transfer operation. J Plast Reconstr Aesthetic Surg 2009;62(11):1510–6.

32. Chim H. Suprafascial radiological characteristics of the superthin profunda artery perforator flap. J Plast Reconstr Aesthetic Surg 2022;75(7): 2064–9.

33. Chim H. Perforator mapping and clinical experience with the superthin profunda artery perforator flap for reconstruction in the upper and lower extremities. J Plast Reconstr Aesthetic Surg 2023;81:60–7.

34. Ahmadzadeh R, Bergeron L, Tang M, et al. The posterior thigh perforator flap or profunda femoris artery perforator flap. Plast Reconstr Surg 2007;119(1): 194–200.

35. Saad A, Sadeghi A, Allen RJ. The anatomic basis of the profunda femoris artery perforator flap: a new option for autologous breast reconstruction—a cadaveric and computer tomography angiogram study. J Reconstr Microsurg 2012;28(06):381–6.

36. Nam YS, Kim HB, Kim SH, et al. Cadaveric Study for Safe Elevation of a Profunda Artery Perforator Flap: Anatomy of the Perforators and Obturator Nerves. J Reconstr Microsurg 2023;39(9):727–33.

37. Lu J, Zhang KK, Graziano FD, et al. Alternative donor sites in autologous breast reconstruction: a clinical practice review of the PAP flap. Gland Surg 2023;12(4):516.

38. Haddock NT, Greaney P, Otterburn D, et al. Predicting perforator location on preoperative imaging for the profunda artery perforator flap. Microsurgery 2012;32(7):507–11.

39. DeLong MR, Hughes DB, Bond JE, et al. A detailed evaluation of the anatomical variations of the profunda artery perforator flap using computed tomographic angiograms. Plast Reconstr Surg 2014; 134(2):186e–92e.

40. Khan UD, Miller J. Reliability of handheld Doppler in planning local perforator–based flaps for extremities. Aesthetic Plast Surg 2007;31:521–5.

41. Taylor GI, Doyle M, McCarten G. The Doppler probe for planning flaps: anatomical study and clinical applications. Br J Plast Surg 1990;43(1):1–16.

42. Heredero S, Sanjuan A, Falguera MI, et al. The thin profunda femoral artery perforator flap for tongue reconstruction. Microsurgery 2020;40(2):117–24.

Thin and Thinned Anterolateral Thigh Flaps for Upper Extremity Reconstruction

Cristin L. Coquillard, MD[a], Jennifer Bai, MD[a], Jason H. Ko, MD, MBA[a,b,*]

KEYWORDS

- Thin ALT flap • Upper extremity reconstruction • Free flap • Microsurgery

KEY POINTS

- The anterolateral thigh (ALT) flap can be elevated in various planes depending on desired thickness of the flap and the reconstructive needs of the defect. The thin ALT flap can be elevated at the superficial fascial plane to achieve a thin, pliable flap.
- For upper extremity reconstruction, thinning the ALT flap primarily or elevating it in the superficial fascial plane vastly improves the aesthetic result and may reduce the number of surgeries required to achieve the final result.
- Both primarily thinning ALT flaps and elevation in the superficial fascial plane are viable options for upper extremity reconstruction with acceptable complication rates.

 Video content accompanies this article at http://www.hand.theclinics.com.

INTRODUCTION

The anterolateral thigh (ALT) flap is a workhorse flap for microsurgical reconstruction. Advantages of the ALT flap include a long vascular pedicle, availability of different tissues, large flap size, good vessel diameter, and minimal donor-site morbidity. The ALT flap was first described by Baek[1] in 1983 and Song[2] in 1984. Originally described as a full-thickness fasciocutaneous flap, the ALT flap can be customized based on individualized reconstructive needs. It can be elevated as a fasciocutaneous, myocutaneous, or adipofascial flap. Moreover, fasciocutaneous ALT flaps can be elevated in different planes of dissection including subfascial, suprafascial, and even thinner planes.

NATURE OF THE PROBLEM

Although the ALT flap can be quite versatile in microsurgical reconstruction, it can vary in adipose thickness based on the plane of elevation and patient habitus. In patients who are more obese, the flap can be bulky due to a thicker layer of subcutaneous tissue. For the subfascial ALT flap, the deep fascia is incised and then the flap is elevated beneath the fascia, which often makes it easier to identify the perforators before they penetrate the fascia.[3] However, the subfascial ALT flap can often be too bulky for the intended reconstructive needs, especially for defects in the upper extremity, which usually require thinner flaps to resurface these defects to allow for adequate function and motion. Other disadvantages of subfascial ALT flaps

[a] Division of Plastic and Reconstructive Surgery, Department of Surgery, Northwestern University Feinberg School of Medicine, Northwestern University, 259 East Erie Street Suite 2060, Chicago, IL 60611, USA;
[b] Department of Orthopaedic Surgery, Northwestern University Feinberg School of Medicine, 259 East Erie Street Suite 2060, Chicago, IL 60611, USA
* Corresponding author. Northwestern Plastic Surgery, 259 East Erie Street, Suite 2060, Chicago, IL 60611.
E-mail address: jason.ko@nm.org

Hand Clin 40 (2024) 199–208
https://doi.org/10.1016/j.hcl.2023.12.001

include donor-site morbidity such as muscle hernia and poor cosmesis if unable to be closed primarily.[4]

Given the differences in the thickness of subcutaneous tissues, there are additional planes of dissection to allow for thinner flaps, such as the thin, super-thin, and ultra-thin ALT flaps. The nomenclature for these is variable in the literature but typically "suprafascial" flaps are elevated just above the crural fascia, whereas "super-thin" are elevated at the level of the superficial fascia within the subcutaneous fat.[5] "Ultra-thin" flaps are elevated through the superficial fat layer.[6] These thinner ALT flaps have decreased flap bulk and provide better contour and pliability, which can help achieve better functional and esthetic outcomes in upper extremity reconstruction.

According to the perforasome concept, the viability of a flap in the superficial fascia plane is derived from perfusion of the perforator as well as the indirect linking vessels connecting to each other.[7] Therefore, a large thin flap can have adequate blood supply to survive even without direct linking vessels, which are found in the deep fat.[4]

A major advantage of a thin ALT flap is improved functional and esthetic outcomes, especially in the setting of extremity reconstruction. Wounds in the upper or lower extremity requiring free tissue transfer benefit from a thin flap that can resurface the extremity rather than just filling a hole.[4] Because range of motion is important for extremity function, soft tissue coverage that is both thin and supple is important for adequate motion underneath. Lin and colleagues state that bulky flaps in the distal upper extremity can impair finger range of motion and decrease hand function.[8] Concerns with the elevation of a thin ALT flap include technical difficulty due to the expertise needed to identify the superficial fascial plane and to dissect and isolate the perforators.[9]

ANATOMY

The vascular pedicle of the ALT flap is the descending branch of the lateral femoral circumflex artery, a branch of the profunda femoral artery, and its venae comitantes, which are found deep between the rectus femoris and vastus lateralis alongside the motor nerve to vastus lateralis. The vessel caliber can be greater than 2 mm, and a pedicle length of 8 to 16 cm can be achieved. The pedicle sends branches to supply the vastus lateralis and rectus femoris flaps, and the overlying skin is supplied by musculocutaneous or septocutaneous perforators. The musculocutaneous pattern comprises the majority of perforators, ranging from 59.2% to 87.1% in previous reports,[3,10–13] despite the original description of the ALT flap as a septocutaneous perforator flap.

The ALT flap is supplied by an average of 2.31 perforators.[10] Although the flap may be taken on multiple perforators, it is not necessary to do so, and the flap may be raised on one perforator alone. The perforators can be quite robust, up to 1 mm in diameter. Only 4 of 405 planned ALTs had perforators too small to elevate a successful flap in a series from Chang Gung Memorial Hospital.[14] In a line drawn between the anterior superior iliac spine (ASIS) to the center of the lateral border of the patella, the cutaneous perforators are concentrated around the halfway point and several centimeters lateral to it, with some also distributed at 33% and 40% the distance of the line.[10,15]

The ALT flap skin is supplied by 2 plexus systems. As the perforator ascends through the subcutaneous tissue perpendicular to the skin, it sends off branches at the level of the deep fascia to form a deep fascial plexus before terminating in the subdermal plexus. These 2 plexus systems are interconnected by small ascending arteries. From the subdermal plexus, recurrent arteries branch deep to supply the underlying subcutaneous tissue.[16]

The relationship between the perforator and the subcutaneous fat is variable, with 3 described types. In type 1, the perforator extends almost perpendicular directly into the subdermal plexus without branching. This comprises 50% of ALT perforators and is the most advantageous for the preservation of blood supply in a thin ALT. In type 2 (35%), perforators branch before reaching the subdermal plexus and extend laterally up to 2 cm, whereas in type 3 (15%), perforators branch shortly after piercing the deep fascia and gradually extend into the subdermal plexus.[17]

PREOPERATIVE PLANNING

Preoperative computed tomography angiograms or formal angiograms may be performed of the lower extremities to elucidate the vascular anatomy of the flap, including the location and caliber of perforators. This may also be used to identify the relationship of the perforators to skin, including how proximally it may branch and how perpendicular it runs. However, in most cases, no imaging of the donor site is necessary, and the flap may be raised "freestyle" or with the use of handheld Doppler to aid in finding perforators.

PREPARATION AND PATIENT POSITIONING

Preoperatively, while in the supine position, the ASIS and the center of the lateral border of the patella are marked. With the patient supine and the foot pointed to the ceiling, a line is drawn between these 2 points. A mark is then placed at the halfway point along this line and at points 5 cm proximal and 5 cm distal to this point. A Doppler is then used to confirm the presence of perforators at these sites. Often, the true location of the perforators is several centimeters lateral to the vertical axis that has been drawn.

PROCEDURAL APPROACH

The defect to be reconstructed is measured and templated onto the skin of the thigh centered around the marked location of the perforators. Under loupe magnification, the medial skin is incised first. The dissection is taken down to the superficial fascial layer that divides the deep and superficial fat. This fascia is akin to the Scarpa's fascia of the abdomen and appears as a white layer that can be quite well defined in some individuals, especially those with high body mass index (BMI). The superficial fascia lies between the larger deep fat globules and the smaller superficial fat globules and may be best seen under tension.[4,18]

Once identified, the flap is elevated laterally in this plane, slowing down as one approaches the axis of the flap in line with the septum between the vastus lateralis and the rectus femoris where the perforators will be found. On locating the perforators, the lateral incision is made, and dissection proceeds similarly from lateral to medial. The best perforator is selected based on size, Doppler signal, and location within the flap. A cuff of fat is left around the perforator as it is traced through the deep fat. The crural fascia is incised longitudinally to allow for dissection of the pedicle proximally. The remainder of the flap elevation proceeds similarly to a standard ALT, dissecting the pedicle through either septum or vastus lateralis, and continuing to the takeoff from the profunda artery or until the desired length is reached.

Alternatively, the flap may be raised in the standard subfascial fashion, starting with the medial incision and dissecting down to the crural fascia. The crural fascia is then incised, and dissection proceeds laterally until the perforators are either identified in the septum or originating from the vastus lateralis. Dissection from the lateral incision then proceeds similarly. The pedicle is skeletonized until its takeoff or the desired length is reached. Before dividing the pedicle proximally, all fat deep to the superficial fascial layer is trimmed off. This is done under loupe magnification, being careful not to overly disrupt the blood supply. An adipofascial cuff of 1 to 2 cm is left around the pedicle. After removing the fat from the deep surface of the flap, the vascular pedicle can be divided, and microvascular anastomoses can be performed in the upper extremity recipient site.

The donor defect is then closed primarily over drains. If the donor site is too wide to close, skin grafts can be used, or a local advancement flap, such as the keystone flap, can be used.[19]

RECOVERY AND REHABILITATION

Postoperatively, the affected portion of the upper extremity is placed in a splint or bulky dressing with strict elevation. The operative splint is removed on postoperative day 5 and replaced with a custom thermoplastic splint. It is imperative that there is no pressure on the flap or the anastomosis and pedicle. Movement of joints that would pull on the anastomosis is avoided for 2 weeks but motion is encouraged immediately postoperatively at other joints, especially the fingers.

CASES

Case 1: A 33-year-old man with a history of intravenous drug use who had necrotizing soft tissue infection of the left dorsal hand and forearm. Following multiple debridements, the wound was appropriate for reconstruction. This resulting defect was reconstructed using a 4 mm thinned ALT flap (**Fig. 1**A–G). This required a great saphenous vein arteriovenous loop to bring the anastomoses outside the zone of injury. The proximal defect, which had only muscle belly rather than tendon exposed, was skin grafted from the thigh.

Fig. 2 demonstrates a bulky postoperative splint that can be used for noncompliant patients in the immediate postoperative period, which elevates the upper extremity while off-loading pressure from the flap and anastomosis. A window in the splint allows for flap monitoring.

Case 2: A 25-year-old man who sustained a crush injury of the left hand at work 2 years before presentation. He had undergone 12 previous surgeries and had developed significant scar contracture of the dorsum of the hand, significantly limiting finger motion. The scar was excised, and extensor tenolysis and metacarpal phalangeal joint capsulotomies were performed followed by placement of TenoGlide (Integra, Princeton, NJ) and reconstruction of the soft tissue defect with a thinned ALT from the right thigh (**Fig. 3**A–G). The patient had a good functional improvement but did require 2 flap debulking procedures, 3 and 6 months after his index flap procedure, demonstrating the challenges of achieving a good contour of the dorsal

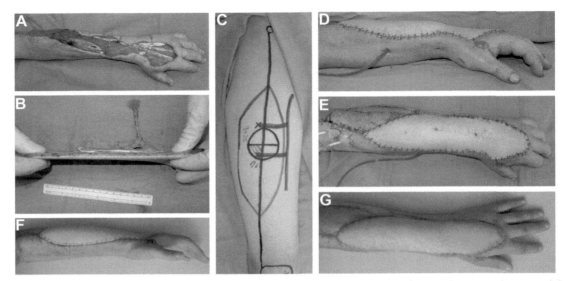

Fig. 1. A 33-year-old man with forearm and hand defect following necrotizing fasciitis due to IV drug use. (*A*) Defect following partial closure with Jacobs ladder and vacuum dressing, (*B*) 4 mm thinned flap based off 2 perforators, (*C*) Marked landmarks and design of the ALT flap, showing axis, pedicle location, perforator location, and flap size of 9 × 25 cm, (*D, E*) immediate postoperative appearance, and (*F, G*) 1-month postoperative appearance.

hand despite aggressive thinning during the flap elevation (**Fig. 4**A–G).

Case 3: A 64-year-old right-hand-dominant woman with history of Hodgkin lymphoma and breast cancer presented after previously having a right forearm mass excised at an outside hospital. Pathology demonstrated a 25 × 15 cm leiomyosarcoma, which had positive margins. She presented to our center for resection of her residual disease. The radial sensory nerve was resected during tumor extirpation, and the resulting defect had multiple extensor tendons exposed. Her forearm was reconstructed using a thinned ALT flap from the left thigh that was neurotized by incorporation of the lateral femoral cutaneous nerve (LFCN, **Fig. 5**A–F). **Fig. 6**A–E demonstrates an excellent contour match at long-term follow-up, at which time she did have sensation in the

neurotized flap. Her wrist and finger range of motion are demonstrated in Video 1.

Case 4: A 25-year-old right-hand-dominant man who had a volar forearm synovial sarcoma resected in Mexico 11 years before presentation, which had recurred. Resection of the tumor left an 11 × 7 cm radial volar forearm defect that included excision of the radial artery. This was reconstructed using a flow-through thin ALT flap based on a single perforator from the right thigh (**Fig. 7**A–E). Video 2 demonstrates good range of motion and contour match at 2-month follow-up.

OUTCOMES AND DISCUSSION

Since its first descriptions in the 1980s by Baek[1] and Song and colleagues,[2] the ALT flap has become a workhorse for many reconstructive

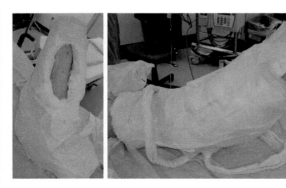

Fig. 2. A splint is placed postoperatively that elevates the extremity, offloads pressure from the flap and anastomosis, and allows for flap monitoring.

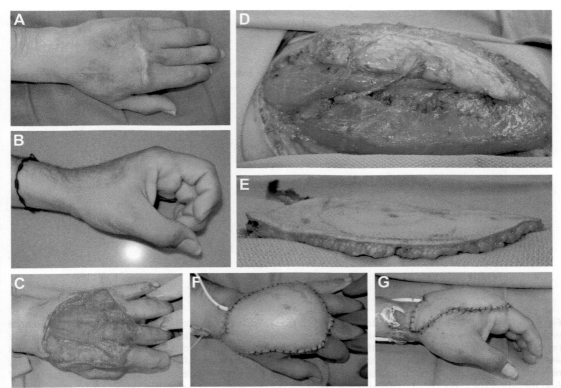

Fig. 3. A 25-year-old male with previous left hand crush injury and scar contracture who underwent scar excision, tenolysis, capsulotomies, and soft tissue reconstruction with thinned ALT. (*A*) Preoperative view of dorsal scar. (*B*) Preoperative maximal finger flexion. (*C*) The resultant defect following scar excision, tenolysis, and placement of TenoGlide. (*D*) Initial thickness of the flap elevated subfascially, demonstrating 2 perforators. (*E*) Final flap thickness after thinning. (*F, G*) Immediate postoperative appearance.

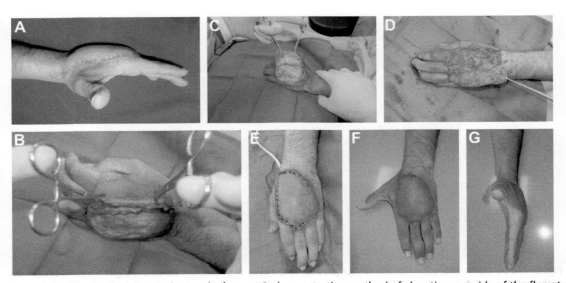

Fig. 4. Debulking and postoperative results for case 2, demonstrating method of elevating one side of the flap at a time to maintain vascularity while debulking. (*A*) Two months after index surgery. (*B, C*) Initial hemiflap debulking. (*D*) Second hemiflap debulking. (*E*) Immediate postoperative results. (*F, G*) One year postoperative follow-up.

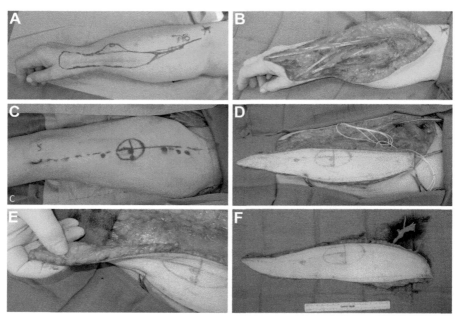

Fig. 5. A 64-year-old woman with history of previously excised leiomyosarcoma of the right forearm presented with evidence of residual disease, which was reconstructed with a neurotized thin ALT flap. (*A*) The planned resection by Orthopedic Oncology of the existing scar and area of residual disease. (*B*) Defect of dorsal forearm and hand after wide resection involving exposed extensor tendons as well as resection of the radial sensory nerve. (*C*) ALT flap design with marking of perforators. (*D*) Elevation of a neurotized free ALT flap. (*E*) ALT flap following thinning. (*F*) ALT flap after harvest with pedicle and LFCN for neurotization.

needs. The ALT flap has many advantages that contribute to its versatility—large maximum size, long and large caliber pedicle, the ability to use as either a free or pedicled flap, and minimal donor-site morbidity.[3] It is traditionally taken as a fasciocutaneous flap, although it may be used as a chimeric flap with vastus lateralis or rectus femoris if extra bulk is needed, or fascia lata for

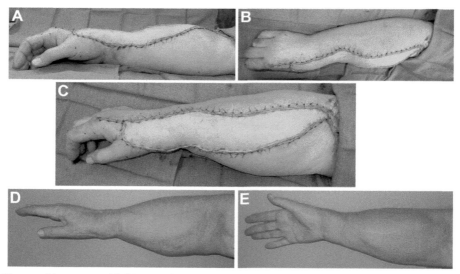

Fig. 6. A 64-year-old woman with history of previously excised leiomyosarcoma of the right forearm presented with evidence of residual disease, which was reconstructed with a neurotized thin ALT flap. (*A–C*) Inset of thinned ALT flap with good contour match with forearm and hand. (*D, E*) Reconstruction with neurotized free ALT flap with LFCN to radial sensory nerve neurotization 10 months postoperatively demonstrating appropriate contour.

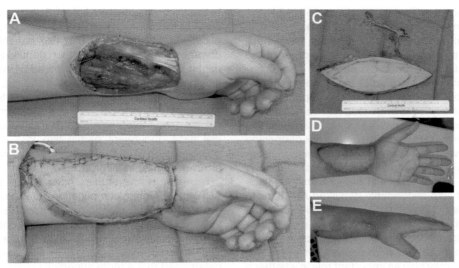

Fig. 7. A 29-year-old man who presented with a synovial sarcoma of his left wrist was reconstructed with a free thin ALT flow through flap to reconstruct the radial artery. (*A*) Resulting defect after resection of left wrist soft tissue sarcoma including resection of radial artery and the radial sensory nerve with exposed muscle and tendon. (*B*) Reconstruction performed with a free thin ALT flow through flap. (*C*) The thin ALT flow through flap was based on a single perforator—the oblique branch of the lateral femoral circumflex artery. (*D, E*) Postoperative result after ALT flow through flap 2 months later.

vascularized tendon reconstruction. Additionally, it may be neurotized via the LFCN.[20] The ALT flap may also be used as a flow-through flap, which is particularly useful in the upper extremity if there are vascular gaps.[3] The flap's ease of dissection is highly variable based on patient anatomy but is quite simple when perforators are septocutaneous. If all perforators course through muscle, however, flap dissection can be tedious unless taken with a cuff of vastus lateralis.

The most significant drawback of using the ALT flap is its potential bulk, which depends on patient habitus. In high BMI patients, the flap can be quite thick. This is particularly an issue with distal upper extremity reconstruction, where the skin and subcutaneous tissue tend to be thin. In an era when microsurgery has advanced enough that we should always consider the esthetics of flap reconstruction and not just flap survival and function, a bulky flap on the upper extremity may be an unacceptable outcome. Recent modifications of the ALT flap have aimed to combat this issue. These include raising it as an adipofascial flap and applying a skin graft, debulking the flap with further surgeries once healed, or creating a thin ALT flap at the time of elevation through dissection in the suprafascial plane or debulking during the index surgery.[21]

The idea of a thinner ALT flap has existed for decades. Koshima and colleagues first described remedying thick flaps by "sacrificing a large amount of fatty tissue" in 1993.[22] In 1996, Kimura and colleagues described a thinned ALT flap through elevation in a plane just superficial to the deep fascia and then defatting the layer of fat deep to the superficial fascia. They left a 1 cm cuff of fat around the perforator. In their series of 5 cases, the final flap thickness ranged from 2 to 5 mm thick. Except for one partial flap loss of the distal flap in an area that was 2 mm thick, the flaps all healed well.[23] Kimura later went on to describe a series of 31 patients using the same technique. In this series, 2 flaps had full thickness partial necrosis, and 7 had superficial necrosis only. They determined the thinned ALT flap was reliable in a 9 cm radius from the perforator and when kept at least 3 mm thick.[17]

Some have questioned whether ALT flap thinning leads to critically reduced flap perfusion. A cadaver injection study by Alkureishi and colleagues demonstrated significantly less dye filling in the distal part of ALT flaps thinned to 3 to 4 mm with a 2 cm fascial cuff around the perforator and almost no dye filling distally in those flaps with a 1 cm fascial cuff.[16] A later cadaver injection study by Nojima and colleagues corroborated these findings, indicating the skin surface vascular territory of thinned ALTs was 83.3% that of standard ALTs. This group also determined the pedicle cuff "danger zone" distances from the pedicle for flap thicknesses of 4, 6, and 8 mm to be 33 to 37 mm, 30 to 35 mm, and 27 to 31, in the cranial-caudal axis, respectively, and 30 to 34 mm, 28 to 31 mm, and 25 to 29 mm in the medial to lateral axis, respectively.[15] Flap thickness evidently plays a role in the safe diameter of the adipofascial cuff around the pedicle.

Although cadaver studies have demonstrated reduced perfusion of thinned ALT flaps, this has not necessarily led to increased flap complications in clinical studies. Cadaver studies of vascular territories are limited by the theoretic lack of opening of choke vessels between perforasomes that occurs in vivo. Cigna and colleagues found no increased complications in primarily thinned flaps compared with secondarily debulked ALT flaps in their series of 45 patients. Additionally, the secondarily debulked flaps required significantly more surgeries to achieve their reconstructive goals than those that were primarily thinned.[24]

Flap size may play an important role in whether a flap will tolerate thinning. A systematic review of 88 flaps among 11 articles showed that flaps larger than 150 cm^2 were significantly more likely to have necrosis (25.93% vs 6.56%). However, this study did not differentiate between partial or full thickness necrosis and the degree to which flaps were thinned.[25] Viviano and colleagues corroborated the safety of primary thinning in a comparison between 53 thinned and subfascial ALTs, including large flaps greater than 240 cm^2. In this study, there were no cases of partial flap necrosis in the thinned group and only one flap loss, due to hematoma.[26]

In 2013, Hong and colleagues described the elevation of the ALT flap at the superficial fascial plane to achieve a thin flap. In their series of 54 flaps, there was only one flap loss (98% survival). Three flaps required subsequent debulking, all in high BMI patients. Notably, those donor sites that required skin grafting had excellent contour compared with the contralateral side, as opposed to traditionally elevated ALTs.[18] This group later expanded their series to 81 thin ALTs. Again, the overall flap survival rate was 98% (2 flap losses). They also reported 5 partial losses (6%) with 2 requiring secondary procedures while the rest healed secondarily.[4] Innocenti later described a hybrid technique of thinning and elevation in the superfascial plane in which the medial aspect of the flap is elevated subfascially, the perforator is identified and protected with a cuff of deep fascia, then the medial flap is thinned and the remaining lateral flap is elevated in the superficial fascial plane. They reported a 100% flap survival rate with 4 out of 16 minor complications.[27]

Seth and Iorio were the first to compare outcomes between suprafascial and "superthin" (elevation in the superficial fascial plane) ALT flaps.

In their retrospective review of 25 patients, there were no instances of partial or total flap loss. Complications were seen in 6 (24%) patients, most commonly the need for further debulking (3 patients).[5] Their group later compared 51 ALT flaps, including 16 subfascial, 23 suprafascial, and 12 superthin (superficial fascial) flaps and found no significant difference in complications. Two (16.7%) superthin and no subfascial or suprafascial flaps underwent partial flap loss. The only complete flap loss was in a subfascial ALT. Flap size was similar in all groups.[28]

However, some studies have shown that thin ALTs have higher complication rates than those elevated in the standard subfascial plane. In 2022, 303 ALTs for lower extremity reconstruction were retrospectively reviewed to assess for risk factors for partial flap loss. In this study, they determined that a more superficial plane of elevation was associated with more partial flap loss, with 25.53% partial loss in the supradeep fat layer (superficial fascial) versus 7.78% partial loss elevated subfascially. It should be noted, however, that the ALT flaps elevated in the supradeep layer were significantly larger than the subfascial flaps and a subgroup analysis could not be performed due to an overall low necrosis rate.[29] Various techniques have been proposed to improve outcomes in thin ALT flaps, including perforator centralization,[30] microdissection,[31] and use of color Doppler ultrasound.[9]

Both primarily thinning ALT flaps and elevation in the superficial fascial plane are viable options for upper extremity reconstruction with acceptable complication rates. The main advantage of thinning following standard elevation in the suprafascial or subfascial plane is the relative ease of dissection. Hong and colleagues did identify a learning curve to raising the flap in the superficial fascial plane.[4] However, in terms of donor-site morbidity, elevation in the superficial fascial plane has the clear advantage with a much less marked contour deformity if skin grafting is necessary. This method may also increase the preservation of thigh sensation through protection of the LFCN that runs in the deep fat.[5]

SUMMARY

Upper extremity reconstruction remains challenging due to the high functional and esthetic demands of this location. The ALT, as a workhorse flap for many types of reconstruction, is an excellent option for the upper extremity. Thinning it primarily or elevating it in the superficial fascial plane vastly improves the esthetic result and may reduce the number of surgeries required to achieve the final result. Although the rate of partial flap necrosis has been shown in some studies to be higher, it is unclear if this bears clinical significance in upper extremity reconstruction and must be weighed against the donor-site morbidity and additional surgeries typically required in standard ALT flaps.

CLINICS CARE POINTS

- The ALT flap can be elevated in various planes depending on desired thickness of the flap and the reconstructive needs of the defect. The thin ALT flap can be elevated at the superficial fascial plane to achieve a thin, pliable flap.
- For upper extremity reconstruction, thinning the ALT flap primarily or elevating it in the superficial fascial plane vastly improves the esthetic result and may reduce the number of surgeries required to achieve the final result.
- Both primarily thinning ALT flaps and elevation in the superficial fascial plane are viable options for upper extremity reconstruction with acceptable complication rates.

DISCLOSURE

J.H. Ko is a consultant for Integra Lifesciences, Inc.; Checkpoint Surgical, Inc.; EDGe Surgical, Inc.; and ImmersiveTouch, Inc. He is also on the Scientific Advisory Board for Mesh Suture, Inc. Otherwise, the authors have nothing to disclose.

SUPPLEMENTARY DATA

Supplementary data related to this article can be found online at https://doi.org/10.1016/j.hcl.2023.12.001

REFERENCES

1. Baek SM. Two new cutaneous free flaps: the medial and lateral thigh flaps. Plast Reconstr Surg 1983;71(3):354–65.
2. Song YG, Chen GZ, Song YL. The free thigh flap: a new free flap concept based on the septocutaneous artery. Br J Plast Surg 1984;37(2):149–59.
3. Wei FC, Jain V, Celik N, et al. Have we found an ideal soft-tissue flap? An experience with 672 anterolateral thigh flaps. Plast Reconstr Surg 2002;109(7):2219–26 [discussion 2227-30].
4. Hong JP, Choi DH, Suh H, et al. A new plane of elevation: the superficial fascial plane for perforator flap elevation. J Reconstr Microsurg 2014;30(7):491–6.
5. Seth AK, Iorio ML. Super-Thin and Suprafascial Anterolateral Thigh Perforator Flaps for Extremity Reconstruction. J Reconstr Microsurg 2017;33(7):466–73.
6. Cha HG, Hur J, Ahn C, et al. Ultra-Thin Anterolateral Thigh Free Flap: An Adipocutaneous Flap with the Most Superficial Elevation Plane. Plast Reconstr Surg 2023. https://doi.org/10.1097/PRS.0000000000010295.
7. Saint-Cyr M, Wong C, Schaverien M, et al. The perforasome theory: vascular anatomy and clinical implications. Plast Reconstr Surg 2009;124(5):1529–44.
8. Lin TS, Jeng SF, Chiang YC. Resurfacing with full-thickness skin graft after debulking procedure for bulky flap of the hand. J Trauma 2008;65(1):123–6.
9. Suh YC, Kim SH, Baek WY, et al. Super-thin ALT flap elevation using preoperative color doppler ultrasound planning: Identification of horizontally running pathway at the deep adipofascial layers. J Plast Reconstr Aesthetic Surg 2022;75(2):665–73.
10. Kimata Y, Uchiyama K, Ebihara S, et al. Anatomic variations and technical problems of the anterolateral thigh flap: a report of 74 cases. Plast Reconstr Surg 1998;102(5):1517–23.
11. Pribaz JJ, Orgill DP, Epstein MD, et al. Anterolateral thigh free flap. Ann Plast Surg 1995;34(6):585–92.
12. Xu DC, Zhong SZ, Kong JM, et al. Applied anatomy of the anterolateral femoral flap. Plast Reconstr Surg 1988;82(2):305–10.
13. Zhou G, Qiao Q, Chen GY, et al. Clinical experience and surgical anatomy of 32 free anterolateral thigh flap transplantations. Br J Plast Surg 1991;44(2):91–6.
14. Wei FC, Jain V, Suominen S, et al. Confusion among perforator flaps: what is a true perforator flap? Plast Reconstr Surg 2001;107(3):874–6.
15. Nojima K, Brown SA, Acikel C, et al. Defining vascular supply and territory of thinned perforator flaps: part I. Anterolateral thigh perforator flap. Plast Reconstr Surg 2005;116(1):182–93.
16. Alkureishi LW, Shaw-Dunn J, Ross GL. Effects of thinning the anterolateral thigh flap on the blood supply to the skin. Br J Plast Surg 2003;56(4):401–8.
17. Kimura N, Satoh K, Hasumi T, et al. Clinical application of the free thin anterolateral thigh flap in 31 consecutive patients. Plast Reconstr Surg 2001;108(5):1197–208 [discussion: 1209-10].
18. Hong JP, Chung IW. The superficial fascia as a new plane of elevation for anterolateral thigh flaps. Ann Plast Surg 2013;70(2):192–5.
19. Turin SY, Spitz JA, Alexander K, et al. Decreasing ALT donor site morbidity with the keystone flap. Microsurgery 2018;38(6):621–6.
20. King EA, Ozer K. Free skin flap coverage of the upper extremity. Hand Clin 2014;30(2):201–9, vi.
21. Friedrich JB, Katolik LI, Vedder NB. Soft tissue reconstruction of the hand. J Hand Surg Am 2009;34(6):1148–55.

22. Koshima I, Fukuda H, Yamamoto H, et al. Free ante-rolateral thigh flaps for reconstruction of head and neck defects. Plast Reconstr Surg 1993;92(3): 421–8 [discussion 429-30].

23. Kimura N, Satoh K. Consideration of a thin flap as an entity and clinical applications of the thin anterolat-eral thigh flap. Plast Reconstr Surg 1996;97(5): 985–92.

24. Cigna E, Minni A, Barbaro M, et al. An experience on primary thinning and secondary debulking of ante-rolateral thigh flap in head and neck reconstruction. Eur Rev Med Pharmacol Sci 2012;16(8):1095–101.

25. Sharabi SE, Hatef DA, Koshy JC, et al. Is primary thinning of the anterolateral thigh flap recommen-ded? Ann Plast Surg 2010;65(6):555–9.

26. Viviano SL, Liu FC, Therattil PJ, et al. Peripheral Pruning: A Safe Approach to Thinning Extra-Large Anterolateral Thigh Flaps. Ann Plast Surg 2018; 80(4 Suppl 4):S164–7.

27. Innocenti M, Calabrese S, Tanini S, et al. A Safer Way to Harvest a Superthin Perforator Flap. Plast Reconstr Surg 2021;147(3):466–9.

28. Diamond S, Seth AK, Chattha AS, et al. Outcomes of Subfascial, Suprafascial, and Super-Thin Anterolat-eral Thigh Flaps: Tailoring Thickness without Added Morbidity. J Reconstr Microsurg 2018;34(3):176–84.

29. Min K, Hong JP, Suh HP. Risk Factors for Partial Flap Loss in a Free Flap: A 12-Year Retrospective Study of Anterolateral Thigh Free Flaps in 303 Lower Ex-tremity Cases. Plast Reconstr Surg 2022;150(5): 1071e–81e.

30. Suh YC, Kim NR, Jun DW, et al. The perforator-centralizing technique for super-thin anterolateral thigh perforator flaps: Minimizing the partial necrosis rate. Arch Plast Surg 2021;48(1):121–6.

31. Liang JL, Liu XY, Qiu T, et al. Microdissected thin an-terolateral thigh perforator flaps with multiple perfo-rators: A series of case reports. Medicine (Baltim) 2018;97(4):e9454.

Evolution and Diversity of Medial Sural Artery Perforator Flap for Hand Reconstruction

Yun-Huan Hsieh, MBBS, MS(PRS)[a,b,1], Hao-I Wei, MD[a,2], Chung-Chen Hsu, MD[a,2], Cheng-Hung Lin, MD, MBA, FACS[a,2],*

KEYWORDS

- Medial sural artery perforator flap • Hand reconstruction • Microsurgery • Mutilated hand

KEY POINTS

- Free medial sural artery perforator (MSAP) flap is a thin, pliable flap with mostly hairless skin.
- Free MSAP flap is versatile for hand and upper limb reconstruction. It can be raised as a simple fasciocutaneous, split-skin-paddle, and chimeric flap.
- Multiple non-vascularized nerve, tendon, and vein grafts can be harvested from the donor site, augmenting the repertoire for complex hand reconstruction.
- Endoscope-assisted perforator identification can enhance the perforator localization and the precision of MSAP flap design.
- If a sizable donor defect is anticipated, the shoelace closure technique should be considered.

INTRODUCTION

Major trauma, infection, and malignancy are the most common etiologies of large complex upper limb defects. From 2006 to 2020, a total of 67 patients underwent upper limb reconstruction using the medial sural artery perforator (MSAP) flap at Chang Gung Memorial Hospital. Sixty-four (95.5%) were caused by trauma, 1 (1.5%) was the result of necrotizing fasciitis, and 2 (3.0%) were due to oncological resection. Sites of defects are summarized in **Fig. 1**.

The reconstruction goal of the distal forearm and hand is primarily focused on resurfacing.[1–3] A selection of pedicled flaps including the posterior interosseous artery flap, reverse radial forearm flap,[4] reverse lateral arm flap,[5] pedicled anterolateral thigh (ALT) flap,[6] and groin flap[6,7] are classical

options. Microsurgery with radial forearm flap, ALT flap,[8,9] and the recently popularized MSAP flap[1,2,10–13] offer greater freedom of inset with diverse tissue components for refined reconstruction of mutilated upper limb defects.

The study of the medial sural artery can be traced back to Manchot in 1889,[14,19] who described "two large arterial branches, sural arteries, emerge at the level of the knee, often from a common stem." The discovery of "cutaneous sural artery branches from the muscular branches of gastrocnemius muscle" can also be attributed to Manchot[14] In 1975, Taylor and colleagues designated the "popliteal flap," an island flap supplied by musculocutaneous branches of the medial and lateral sural vessels.[15] The angiosomes of MSAP were subjected to further study by Taylor.[16] Similarly, Mathes and Vasconez described

[a] Department of Plastic and Reconstructive Surgery, Chang Gung Memorial Hospital, Chang Gung Medical College and Chang Gung University, Taoyuan, Taiwan; [b] Department of Plastic and Reconstructive Surgery, St. Vincent Private Hospital, East Melbourne, Australia
[1] Present address: 512/51 Thistlethwaite Street, South Melbourne, Victoria, Australia.
[2] Present address: No. 5, Fuxing St., Guishan Dist., Taoyuan City 333, Taiwan (R.O.C.).
* Corresponding author. No. 5, Fuxing Street, Guishan District, Taoyuan City 333, Taiwan (R.O.C.)
E-mail address: lukechlin@gmail.com

Hand Clin 40 (2024) 209–220
https://doi.org/10.1016/j.hcl.2023.08.008
0749-0712/24/© 2023 Elsevier Inc. All rights reserved.

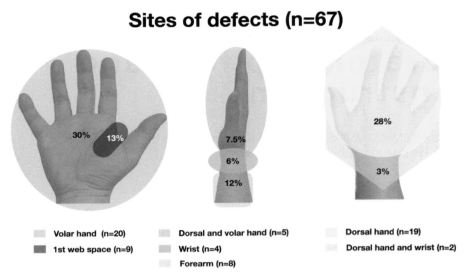

Sites of defects (n=67)

30% 13%

7.5%

6%

12%

28%

3%

Volar hand (n=20)   Dorsal and volar hand (n=5)   Dorsal hand (n=19)
1st web space (n=9)   Wrist (n=4)   Dorsal hand and wrist (n=2)
Forearm (n=8)

Fig. 1. Summary of defect sites.

the use of the "medial skin-fascial gastrocnemius flap" based on medial gastrocnemius musculocutaneous perforators in 1982,[17] which was later named the sural flap in 1997.[18] In 2001, Hallock demonstrated the potential for the design of a "gastrocnemius perforator-based flap" based on an anatomic study of above knee amputation specimens.[11,19] Cavadas and colleagues presented the first free MSAP flap series for lower limb reconstruction in the same year. In the same article, the flap was officially named.[20]

The flourishing interest in the MSAP flap is reflected in recent publications. Each report showcases the diversity and application of the flap. With the accumulated collateral experience of the MSAP flap and advanced understanding of its surgical anatomy and variations, the MSAP flap can now be considered a safe workhorse flap for extremity and head and neck reconstruction.[3,11,19–27] The free MSAP flap is a thin and pliable flap with predictable vascular anatomy and good pedicle length (8–12 cm).[1,3,26] It typically allows reconstruction of small to medium size defects,[1,26] However, a large MSAP flap of $20 \times 10 \text{ cm}^2$ in size was reported previously.[3] It can be raised as a fasciocutaneous flap or a chimeric flap with the inclusion of the medial gastrocnemius muscle.[26,27] In the presence of 2 or more perforators, a split MSAP flap with 2 or more separate skin paddles can also be applied for complex multifaceted non-elliptical defect reconstruction.[28] These versatile features have heightened the suitability of MSAP flaps for complex hand reconstruction. The texture, color, and contour of the medial calf are reasonably matched

with the forearm and hand; therefore, a good outcome following the reconstruction can be achieved.[1] The flap can be raised with deep fascia and provides a gliding surface for the (reconstructed) tendon. The ability to harvest isolated tendon/nerve/vein grafts from the same donor site further broadens the armamentarium for functional reconstruction of composite defects of the hand.[1,3,11,26]

NATURE OF THE COMPLEX HAND DEFECTS

- Mutilated upper limbs are commonly associated with major trauma, and patients should be stabilized before attending to the management of upper limb trauma.
- Complex hand injuries are grossly contaminated and associated with composite tissue loss.
- Locoregional flaps may be unavailable in major hand trauma.
- Functional and aesthetic outcomes are equally crucial for hand reconstruction.

ANATOMY
Medial Sural Artery Anatomy

The medial sural artery (MSA) either originates from the middle one-third of the popliteal artery (PA) or bifurcates from a shared common stem with the lateral sural artery from the popliteal artery at the level of the femoral condyle.[11,19,29] The MSA exits the popliteal fossa between the 2 heads of the gastrocnemius accompanied by the medial sural cutaneous nerve.[14] The MSA then travels

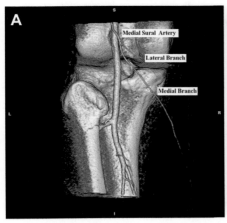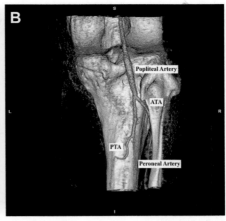

Fig. 2. Bilateral lower limb computed tomography angiography from the same patient showed different medial sural artery (MSA) branching patterns. (*A*) Left leg: Type II (medial and lateral branch). (*B*) Right leg: Type IV (unfavorable anatomy for medial sural artery perforator [MSAP] flap, no medial sural artery identified).

posteriorly (superficially) and enters the medial gastrocnemius at the knee joint level. Subsequently, the MSA courses and branches within the medial gastrocnemius muscle rather superficially with a depth ranging from 1.3 ± 0.4 cm to 0.5 ± 0.2 cm.[30]

The medial gastrocnemius muscle is classically defined as a Type I muscle based on the Mathes and Nahai Classification. However, within the medial gastrocnemius, several branching patterns have been described and classified by Dusseldorp and colleagues (Type I: Single dominant MSA branch; Type II: Dual dominant MSA branches; Type III: Three or more branches).[30] In addition, the authors proposed a Type IV pattern where no MSA branch is detectable from computed tomography angiography (CTA). Similar to Dusseldorp's findings,[30] the authors found the Type II pattern is the most prevalent, followed by Type I and Type III. Only 4% of the lower limb CTAs showed no detectable MSA branch to the medial gastrocnemius muscle (unpublished data) compared with 10% in the published literature.[13,30] Some patients displayed different MSA branching patterns in their bilateral lower limb CTA (**Fig. 2**).

In addition to MSA branches, the muscle also receives blood supply from vascular connection with the lateral head, the muscular branch of the posterior tibial artery (PTA), and the peroneal artery (PA). Based on these clinical observations, the medial gastrocnemius muscle is more commonly a Mathes and Nahai Type V and Type II muscle than a Type I.

Medial Sural Artery Perforator Flap Anatomy

The MSA is the dominant artery supplying the medial gastrocnemius muscle. The caliber of the MSA at its origin ranges from 1 to 4 mm[23,29] and abruptly reduces after its bifurcation.[1,3,26,29] The dominant venae comitantes (VC) is significantly larger than the MSA and is up to 5 mm.[11] The MSA has a pure intramuscular course and provides a 8 to 12 cm pedicle length for the MSAP flap.[1] The MSA gives rise to 1 to 3 cutaneous perforators (mean = 1.2) located between 8 and 13 cm (78.2%) below the popliteal fossa in this case series (**Fig. 3, Table 1**). This echoes the finding from Kim and colleagues,[21] who stated that the majority of the perforators can be found at 8 cm from the midpoint of the popliteal crease within the distal half circle down with a radius of 2 cm. The perforators commonly follow a short "lazy-S" course in the areolar tissue to supply the overlying skin.[19–21] Hence, there is poor correlation between perforator Doppler signals and the actual perforator locations. The perforators in the medial sural territory are not always derived from the MSA. Three cases (4.5%) of the anatomic variant were identified, where the PTA was the source of these perforators.

PREOPERATIVE PLANNING
Recipient Site Evaluation

- In cases of traumatic injuries of the upper limb, principles of early management of severe trauma should be followed.
- Judicious debridement and detailed tissue component evaluation of the composite defect are vital for successful upper extremity reconstruction.
- The wound bed needs to be infection-free, and the oncological resection margin should be cleared before the reconstruction.

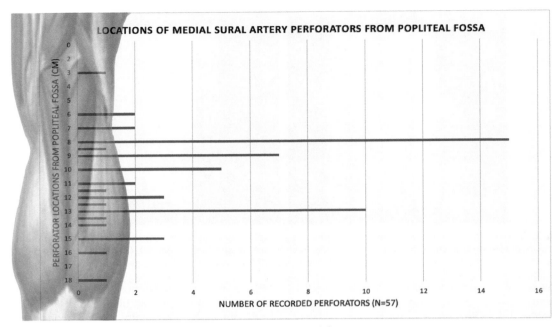

Fig. 3. Summary of detected MSAP locations from the popliteal fossa.

- CTA/magnetic resonance angiography (MRA)/ angiogram may be required to assess suitable recipient vessels in major traumatic defects of the upper limb.

Medial Sural Artery Perforator Flap Donor Evaluation

- Obtain history and inspect bilateral lower limbs for concurrent injury and scars from previous operations.

Table 1
Versatility of medial sural artery perforator flap for upper extremity reconstruction

Flap Harvest Variations		Number of Cases (%)
Numbers of perforators	1	56 (83.6%)
	2	9 (13.4%)
	3	2 (3.0%)
Large skin paddle (>100 cm²)		5 (7.5%)
Split skin paddle		1 (1.5%)
Chimeric flap (with medial gastrocnemius muscle)		4 (6.0%)
Plantaris tendon		12 (17.9%)
Split Achilles tendon		1 (1.5%)
Sural nerve		4 (6.0%)
Saphenous nerve		3 (4.5%)

- In the presence of concurrent trauma to the proximal tibia or medial calf, the use of the MSAP flap is contraindicated.
- Skin pinch test over the medial calf is performed to assess the thickness of fasciocutaneous tissue and maximal flap width for primary closure.
- Bilateral leg CTA is routinely used for vascular mapping and to assess vascular injuries and variations.
- The donor leg is chosen based on the more favorable MSA anatomy for the determined flap design.
- Similar to harvesting palmaris longus tendon, 5.8% to 31%[31–33] of plantaris may be absent. Split Achilles tendon provides a good alternative option.[1]

SURGICAL PREPARATION AND PATIENT POSITIONING

- Marking: A line is drawn from the midpoint of the popliteal fossa to the medial malleolus. Perforators are located by handheld Doppler centered at the marked line over the midcalf.
- Patients lie in a supine position with the hip abducted and externally rotated and the knee in 90° of flexion (flamingo position).
- Above the knee, a tourniquet is applied and set at 300 mm Hg.
- A stack of sterile towels is placed beneath the lateral compartment of the leg. This supports

the medial calf and stabilizes the operating field.

SURGICAL APPROACH
Endoscope-Assisted Perforator Identification

- Tourniquet-controlled procedure.
- One cm incision over the anterior border of medial gastrocnemius muscle.
- Endoscope: 4 mm diameter, 30-degree endoscope.
- The endoscope is gently introduced into the space between the subcutaneous tissue and deep fascia in the areolar tissue.
- Identify all the available perforators in the territory.
- Corrective markings are made on the skin over the corresponding perforators.

Endoscope-assisted perforator identification addresses the discrepancy between handheld Doppler marking and the actual perforator location due to the "lazy-S" perforator course in the areolar tissue. The corrected perforator mapping increases the flap design safety and reduces donor site morbidity. It is particularly useful when a small or split flap is required. Alternatively, high-definition ultrasound mapping of MSAP also offers an efficacious approach to this clinical challenge.[34]

Fasciocutaneous and Split Medial Sural Artery Perforator Flap Harvest

- The flap is designed based on the defect size, the Doppler-detected perforator location, and the required pedicle length.
- The flap is oriented obliquely along the Langer's line to facilitate primary closure.
- The flap is typically planned between 8 and 13 cm from the center of the popliteal fossa, where most perforators are found.
- Endoscope-assisted perforator identification (optional).
- Harvest begins with an anterior incision (anterior approach) down to the deep fascia.
- Careful exploration in the subfascial plane for cutaneous perforators.
- The flap is re-designed if the locations of the perforators significantly deviate from the Doppler-assisted marking.
- Retrograde tracing of the selected perforator(s) through intramuscular dissection toward the popliteal fossa.
- Gentle dissection and tissue handling are critical to prevent arterial spasm.
- The posterior incision is kept till the final step to prevent accidental traction injury, kinking,

or twisting of the perforators during the dissection.[1]
- Indocyanine green(ICG) fluoroscopy imaging (SPY Fluorescence technology) is used routinely to assess the viability of the donor muscle and flap circulation prior to pedicle ligation.
- In split skin paddle flap design, more than 2 perforators need to be identified and traced. The flap circulation of each paddle is checked post-division before pedicle ligation.

Chimeric Medial Sural Artery Perforator Flap Harvest

- Chimeric MSAP flaps are indicated in hand reconstruction for dead space obliteration, bone and hardware coverage, and soft tissue augmentation.
- The muscle component of the chimeric MSAP flap is either based on the medial branch or the distal runoff of the lateral branch.
- To increase the freedom of the inset, 1 to 2 cm of vascular pedicle proximal to the muscular component of the flap is preferred.

Nonvascularized Grafts Harvesting Through Medial Sural Artery Perforator Flap Donor Site

- Tendon, nerve, and vein grafts are frequently needed in mutilated complex defects of the hand.
- Plantaris tendon can be found between the medial gastrocnemius and soleus muscle over the anterior border of the donor site.
- In the absence of plantaris tendon, a split Achilles tendon can be harvested instead.
- The saphenous nerve and great saphenous vein can be harvested at the anterior border of the donor site. The sural nerve and lesser saphenous vein can be harvested through the posterior border.
- Raising the MSAP flap with the fascial layer provides a gliding surface over the tendons of the hand.

RECOVERY & REHABILITATION

- The patient is monitored in the microsurgery intensive care unit (Micro ICU) for 3 to 5 days. Frequent and systematic flap monitoring is essential.
- The flap is monitored by serial clinical assessments. Laser Doppler perfusion imaging (LDPI),[35] and a newly developed machine learning application[36] have also been trialed.

Table 2
Summary and outcomes of medial sural artery perforator flap for upper extremity reconstruction

Indications		Number of Cases
Etiology of defect	Trauma	64 (95.5%)
	Infection	2 (3.0%)
	Oncological resection	1 (1.5%)
Microvascular re-exploration	Arterial insufficiency	3 (4.5%)
	Venous Congestion	5 (7.5%)
	Mixed	1 (1.5%)
	Flap salvaged	7 (77.8%)
Flap outcomes	Successful flap	65 (97.0%)
	Failed flap	2 (3.0%)
Donor site managements	Primary closure	54 (80.6%)
	Shoelace closure	9 (13.4%)
	Skin graft	4 (6.0%)

- Urgent re-exploration is initiated if signs of arterial insufficiency or venous congestion are detected.
- Splint applied to protect the repaired tendons, nerves, and vascular anastomoses.
- Patients are referred to a hand therapist and physiotherapist to initiate the rehabilitation.

OUTCOMES
Medial Sural Artery Perforator Flap Details and Outcome

Sixty-seven patients were identified with an average age of 37.9. The average follow-up period was 16.3 months. The average flap size was 10.6×5.2 cm^2 (range: 3.0×3.0–16×18 cm^2) with an average pedicle length of 9.2 cm (range: 6.0–13.5 cm). There were 5 flaps with a size greater than 100 cm^2, all of which were recovered without complications. Thirty-six (53.7%) used endoscope-assisted perforator identification. Sixty-two fasciocutaneous flaps, 1 split flaps,

and 4 chimeric flaps were utilized in this series (see **Table 1**). Fasciocutaneous flaps were utilized for resurfacing, split skin paddled flaps were used for multifaceted defects, and chimeric flaps were used for dead space obliteration and tissue augmentation.

Twelve plantaris tendons were harvested for flexor pollicis longus, flexor tendons of the forearm, lateral band, and extensor digitorum communis (EDC) reconstructions. One patient required both plantaris tendon and split Achilles tendon for EDC III and EDC II reconstruction, respectively. Seven nerve grafts were harvested through donor sites in this series, including 4 sural nerves and 3 saphenous nerves for median nerve and digital nerve reconstruction. The commonly selected recipient vessels included the radial and ulnar arteries. Digital arteries were also used in 6 cases. Cephalic and dorsal veins were frequently chosen as recipient veins. Alternative recipient veins used were basilic and radial artery VC.

The flap success rate was 97.0%. Nine patients (13.4%) required microvascular re-exploration, 5 due to venous congestion, 3 caused by arterial insufficiency, and 1 had a mixed presentation. Among those needing re-exploration, 7 flaps were successfully salvaged (77.8%), 2 failed flaps were caused by arterial insufficiency and a mixed dysfunction of both artery and vein (**Table 2**).

Donor Site Outcome

The majority of the donor sites were directly closed (80.6%): Nine cases were closed with the shoelace technique (13.4%), and 4 patients (6.0%) had skin grafts (see **Table 2**). The average flap size permissible was 48.5 ± 21.85 cm^2 for primary closure, 94.9 ± 28.13 cm^2 for shoelace closure, and 71.3 ± 37.32 cm^2 for skin graft reconstruction (**Table 3**). Two patients from the primary closure group received donor site scar revision subsequently. One skin-grafted patient needed donor wound debridement and reconstruction with an advancement flap. The flap size in the nonprimary closure group (shoelace + skin graft group) was 39.1 cm^2 (95% CI = 18.2–60.0;

Table 3
Donor site management

Method of Donor Site Closure	Average Flap Length (cm)	Average Flap Width (cm)	Average Flap Size (cm^2)
Primary closure (n = 54)	9.8 ± 3.31	4.8 ± 1.06	48.5 ± 21.85
Shoelace (n = 9)	14.0 ± 2.87	6.7 ± 0.87	94.9 ± 28.13
Skin graft (n = 4)	12.3 ± 3.30	5.5 ± 2.38	71.3 ± 43.09

Table 4
Comparative 2-tailed t-test analysis of medial sural artery perforator flap dimensions and donor site closure methodologies

Method of Donor Site Closure	Flap Length (cm) P-Value (2 Tailed)	Flap Width (cm) P-Value (2 Tailed)	Flap Size (cm^2) P-Value (2 Tailed)
Primary closure vs Shoelace	<0.05	<0.05	<0.05
Primary closure vs Skin graft	0.233	0.597	0.371
Primary closure vs Non-primary closure	<0.05	<0.05	<0.05
Shoelace vs Skin graft	0.400	0.404	0.369

$P < .05$) larger than the primary closure group. The shoelace closure technique could manage a donor defect 23.6 cm^2 larger than the skin graft group (95% CI = −87.7–40.5; $P = .37$). The donor defect in the skin graft group was marginally 22.7 cm^2 larger (95% CI = −45.0–90.4; $P = .04$) than those with primary closure (**Table 4**).

Previously, we have deduced that the width of the flap design is the major determinant for primary closure of the donor site and should be confined within 6 cm.[1,3,26,27] This is reflected in the flap dimensions in this series. Except for the shoelace group, most flaps (85.7%) were designed with a width less than 6 cm. Surprisingly, comparing skin graft and primary closure groups, the flap dimensions were not significantly different ($P = .6$), and their respective flap widths were less than 6 cm on average. This finding reinforced the importance of the skin pinch test when assessing the suitability of the MSAP flap donor site.[37] Patients with well-developed calves or with higher body mass index (BMI) may reduce the permissibility for primary donor site closure.

The statistical analysis highlights the role of the shoelace closure technique in donor site management. It enables the eventual closure of donor sites larger than those reconstructed with skin grafts. This shows that shoelace closure is a valuable

technique in managing sizable donor defects and should be considered before the use of skin graft (**Fig. 4**).

Routine ICG assessment of the medial gastrocnemius muscle showed no devascularization of the retained muscle (**Fig. 5**). This demonstrates that the viability of the muscle can be retained with careful intramuscular dissection and patient selection. Testsonis[38] described the presence of communicating arterioles between medial and lateral gastrocnemius muscles, the musculocutaneous and muscular perforators from soleus, PA, PTA, the remaining MSA branch(es), and the retrograde flow from the retained musculocutaneous perforators which can adequately supply the medial gastrocnemius muscle post dissection.

Despite most donor sites recovering uneventfully, donor site morbidity remains a concern. Kao and colleagues reported self-limiting donor leg weakness worsened with climbing and walking downstairs.[39] In our patient-reported survey, donor site dissatisfaction derives from intermediate functional decline, pain, and scar appearance. However, fundamental function in the donor lower limb was unaffected. This dissatisfaction is more prominent among younger patients and patients needing a higher lower limb functional level (unpublished data).

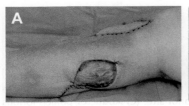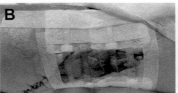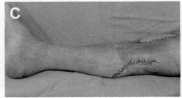

Fig. 4. MSAP flap donor site management with shoelace closure device. (*A*) Partial closure of unopposable donor site. (*B*) Wound management with shoelace closure device (EZip, Taiwan). (*C*) Achieved complete wound closure within 1 week.

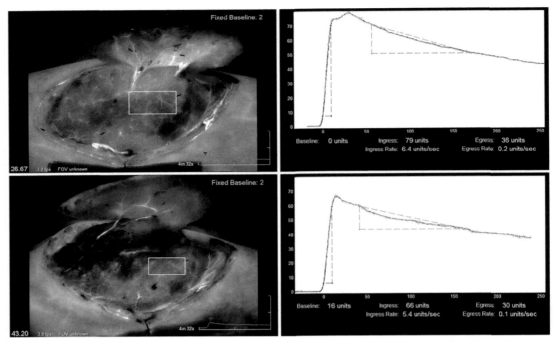

Fig. 5. Intraoperative indocyanine green (ICG) fluorescence angiography of the donor site showing well vascularized medial gastrocnemius muscle post flap harvest. (*Upper*) before intramuscular dissection. (*Lower*) after skeletonizing the vascular pedicle.

Bailout Options

One of the constant challenges of raising perforator flaps is the variation of the perforator distributions and locations. Similar to the experience with the ALT flap, the MSAP may be absent.[3] Although rarely encountered, the posterior tibial artery perforator (PTAP) flap can be the bailout option.

The vascular pedicle of the PTAP flap lies between the flexor digitorum longus and soleus muscle, which is accessible through the same donor site.

As part of anatomic variations, not all perforators identified in the MSA territories are traced back to the MSA. Uncommonly, these perforators are derived from the PTA instead. If this scenario is encountered intraoperatively, the "freestyle" free

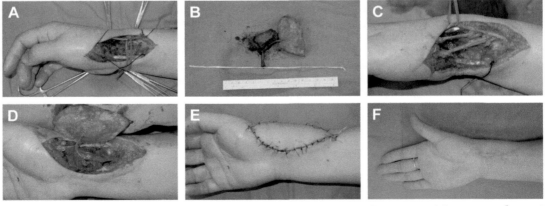

Fig. 6. (*A*) Composite defect at the right radial wrist. (*B*) Chimeric MSAP flap (skin paddle 9 × 5 cm²; muscle 4.5 × 4 cm²) and plantaris tendon graft were harvested from the same donor site. (*C*) Abductor pollicis longus and extensor pollicis brevis reconstructed with plantaris tendon graft. (*D*) Dead space obliterated with muscle component of the flap. (*E*) Fasciocutaneous component for skin defect reconstruction. (*F*) Three-year follow-up showed an acceptable aesthetic outcome without revision surgery.

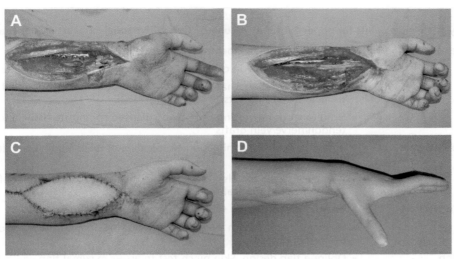

Fig. 7. (*A*) Large left forearm defect with segmental median nerve defect post debridement. (*B*) Sural nerve graft harvest for median nerve reconstruction. (*C*) MSAP flap for soft tissue defect reconstruction with adequate contouring. (*D*) Good functional and aesthetic recovery was achieved at 9-month follow-up after median nerve neurolysis and Bunnell opponensplasty.

flap harvesting concept proposed by Wei and Mardini[40] should be followed.

SECONDARY AND REVISION PROCEDURES

The common secondary procedures post hand and forearm reconstructions with MSAP flaps were debulking (n = 22), tenolysis (n = 20), and tendon transfer (n = 8). Debulking procedures were performed on the volar hand (n = 8), dorsal hand (n = 10), first web space (n = 3), and wrist

(n = 1). To maximize thinning of the flap in a single procedure, a combined excision (<50% of the flap circumference) and liposuction technique was used. About one-third of patients with volar and first web space defects required debulking procedures. This may allow a closer contour match of the MSAP flap to these recipient sites, particularly for glabrous hand reconstruction.

Other recorded revision procedures in this series include 3 minor wound debridements, skin grafting to the hand and forearm (n = 3), and a

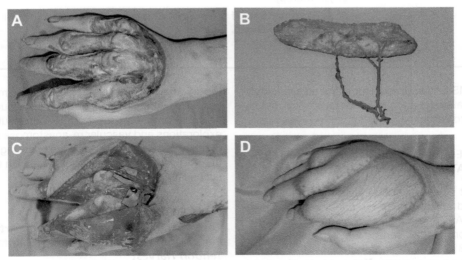

Fig. 8. (*A*) Extensive right dorsal hand defect with exposed bones and joints. (*B*) Three perforators were identified with an endoscope-assisted approach. (*C*) Split skin paddle MSAP flap improved the freedom of the flap inset. (*D*) Uneventful wound healing.

Box 1
Summary of surgical pearls for upper extremity reconstruction with medial sural artery perforator flap

Attributes of the Flap	• Thin and Pliable fasciocutaneous Tissue, less Affected by BMI
	• Less hair-bearing skin compared with other lower limb donor sites
	• Provides a good alternative flap for radial forearm flap, suitable for small to medium size defects
	• Simultaneous harvesting of non-vascularised composite tissue, including tendon/nerve/vein grafts
Patient preparation	• In flamingo position: hip abduction and external rotation; knee flexion at 90°
	• A stack of sterile towels is placed under the lateral compartment of the leg to stabilize the surgical field
Vascular dissection	• Tourniquet-controlled subfascial perforator dissection
	• Perforator exploration via a short anterior incision. Consider endoscope-assisted approach
Flap Design	• Oblique flap design. Skin pinch test to assess maximal flap width (<6 cm) for primary closure
	• It can be raised as a chimeric flap for dead space obliteration
	• It can be raised with a split skin paddle design if 2 or more perforators are present
Pedicle dissection	• Pedicle length 8–12 cm
	• The pedicle length and arterial caliber are sufficient for upper limb reconstruction
	• Trace the pedicle proximal to the bifurcation of the medial and lateral branch to increase the arterial caliber
	• Proximal pedicle dissection also increases venous caliber, which invariably increases the size mismatch
	• Consider using a venous side branch, or ligate the vein more distally to reduce the size mismatch
Donor site	• Less desirable donor scar worsened with a skin graft
	• Self-limiting donor leg weakness on exertion, likely resolve with physiotherapy
	• Consider other flaps if the patient requires a high level of lower limb function, for example, athletes

case of MSAP flap division for acquired syndactyly in preparation for a toe to hand transfer for middle finger reconstruction.

MANAGEMENT OF MEDIAL SURAL ARTERY PERFORATOR FLAP COMPLICATIONS

The most time-critical operative management for hand and distal forearm reconstruction with a free MSAP flap is flap salvage through re-exploration. In this series, the flap salvage rate was 77.8%, which contributed to the overall 97.0% flap success rate. The essence of a good salvage and flap success rate is intense and systematic monitoring by the experienced staff in the Micro ICU, the dedicated ICU for microsurgery. This safety net is highlighted by 2 successful flap salvage cases after 3 consecutive re-explorations and vascular re-anastomoses. Unfortunately, 2 free MSAP flaps were unsalvageable. A free ALT flap was used in each case with eventual successful hand reconstruction.

CLINICAL CASES
Case 1: Free Chimeric Medial Sural Artery Perforator Flap with Concurrent Plantaris Tendon Harvest

A 38-year-old female presented postradical excision of Grade II synovial sarcoma. The radial artery, extensor pollicis brevis (EPB), and abductor pollicis longus (APL) were sacrificed for oncological clearance (**Fig. 6**A). A chimeric MSAP flap was harvested with 22-cm plantaris tendon graft to obliterate the dead space and reconstruct APL and EPB (**Fig. 6**B–E). The radial artery stump and cephalic and dorsal vein were used as recipient vessels. She had an uncomplicated recovery with an acceptable wrist contour (**Fig. 6**F).

Case 2: Free Medial Sural Artery Perforator Flap with Concurrent Sural Nerve Graft Harvest

An 18-year-old female was admitted after falling 10 m. She sustained open Gustilo type IIIB radius and ulna fractures and was referred for a left wrist defect after multiple wound debridements. Composite left wrist defect consisted of ruptured flexor digitorum superficialis (FDS) to the index finger, segmental median nerve loss, and soft tissue defect (**Fig. 7**A). FDS was primarily repaired. A free MSAP flap (10×6 cm^2) was raised for soft tissue coverage, and sural nerve graft was harvested for median nerve reconstruction (**Fig. 7**B, C). She required left median nerve neurolysis and Bunnell opponensplasty 5 months later with good recovery (**Fig. 7**D).

Case 3: Free Split Medial Sural Artery Perforator Flap

A 22-year-old male with epilepsy and intellectual disability presented with a scald burn resulting in a composite right dorsal hand defect (**Fig. 8**A). Three perforators were identified by endoscope-assisted technique. Free MSAP flap was harvested with split skin paddles (13×5 cm^2 and 7×5 cm^2) (**Fig. 8**B). Each skin paddle was reoriented to match the shape of the right dorsal hand defect (**Fig. 8**C). Temporary arthrodesis with K-wire (index to little finger) was performed, immobilization of the fingers in a safe position for flap protection. The postoperative recovery was uneventful (**Fig. 8**D) (**Box 1**).

CLINICS CARE POINTS

- Endoscope-assisted perforator identification is fast, safe, and reliable. It increases the precision of flap design and reduces donor morbidity.
- Oblique flap orientation to facilitate primary donor closure.

- The incidence of venous congestion is higher than arterial insufficiency in free MSAP flaps.
- MSAP pedicle is vulnerable to arterial spasm and is challenging to manage.
- Intensive postoperative flap monitoring and early re-exploration are essential for successful flap salvage.
- Consider the shoelace technique for the large donor site (>6 cm width).

DISCLOSURE

Dr C.-H. Lin is the co-inventor of EZip, the refined shoelace wound closure device, for donor site management in the presented case series.

REFERENCES

1. Lin CH, Lin CH, Lin YT, et al. The medial sural artery perforator flap: A versatile donor site for hand reconstruction. J Trauma 2011;70(3):736–43.
2. Chen SL, Chen TM, Lee CH. Free medial sural artery perforator flap for resurfacing distal limb defects. J Trauma 2005;58(2):323–7.
3. Deek NFAL, Hsiao JC, Do NT, et al. The medial sural artery perforator flap: Lessons learned from 200 consecutive cases. Plast Reconstr Surg 2020; 146(5):630e–41e.
4. Naalla R, Chauhan S, Dave A, et al. Reconstruction of post-traumatic upper extremity soft tissue defects with pedicled flaps: An algorithmic approach to clinical decision making. Chin J Traumatol 2018;21(6): 338–51.
5. Kostakoglu N, Keçik A. Upper Limb Reconstruction with Reverse Flaps. Ann Plast Surg 1997;39(4): 381–9.
6. Zelken JA, Chang NJ, Wei FC, et al. The combined ALT-groin flap for the mutilated and degloved hand. Injury 2015;46(8):1591–6.
7. Abdelrahman M, Zelken J, Huang RW, et al. Suprafascial dissection of the pedicled groin flap: A safe and practical approach to flap harvest. Microsurgery 2018;38(5):458–65.
8. Pederson WC. Upper extremity microsurgery. Plast Reconstr Surg 2001;107(6):1524–43.
9. Hsu CC, Lin YT, Lin CH, et al. Immediate emergency free anterolateral thigh flap transfer for the mutilated upper extremity. Plast Reconstr Surg 2009;123(6): 1739–47.
10. Xie RG, Gu JH, Gong YP, et al. Medial sural artery perforator flap for repair of the hand. J Hand Surg Eur 2007;32(5):512–7.
11. Hallock GG. The Medial Sural Artery Perforator Flap: A Historical Trek from Ignominious to Workhorse. Arch Plast Surg 2022;49(2):240–52.

12. Jeevaratnam JA, Nikkhah D, Nugent NF, et al. The medial sural artery perforator flap and its application in electrical injury to the hand. J Plast Reconstr Aesthetic Surg 2014;67(11):1591–4.

13. Wang X, Mei J, Pan J, et al. Reconstruction of distal limb defects with the free medial sural artery perforator flap. Plast Reconstr Surg 2013;131(1):95–105.

14. Morain WD. [Translator], Manchot C.: The cutaneous arteries of the human body [introduction]. New York, NY: Springer- Verlag; 1983. p. 112.

15. Taylor GI, Daniel RK. The anatomy of several free flap donor sites. Plast Reconstr Surg 1975;56(3): 243–53.

16. Taylor GI, Pan WR. Angiosomes of the leg: Anatomic study and clinical implications. Plast Reconstr Surg 1998;102(3):599–616.

17. Mathes SJ, Vasconez LO. Lower extremity reconstruction. In: Mathes SJ, Nahai F, editors. Clinical applications for muscle and musculocutaneous flaps. St. Louis, MO: CV Mosby Co; 1982. p. 552–3.

18. Mathes SJ, Nahai F. Leg: sural artery flap. In: Reconstructive Surgery: Principles, Anatomy, & Technique2. New York, NY: Churchill Livingstone; 1997. p. 1489–99.

19. Hallock GG. Anatomic basis of the gastrocnemius perforator-based flap. Ann Plast Surg 2001;47(5): 517–22.

20. Cavadas PC, Sanz-Giménez-Rico JR, Gutierrez-de la Cámara A, et al. The medial sural artery perforator free flap. Plast Reconstr Surg 2001;108(6):1609–17.

21. Kim HH, Jeong JH, Seul JH, et al. New design and identification of the medial sural perforator flap: an anatomical study and its clinical applications. Plast Reconstr Surg 2006;117(5):1609–18.

22. Okamoto H, Sekiya I, Mizutani J, et al. Anatomical basis of the medial sural artery perforator flap in Asians. Scand J Plast ReConstr Surg Hand Surg 2007;41(3):125–9.

23. Thione A, Valdatta L, Buoro M, et al. The medial sural artery perforators: anatomic basis for a surgical plan. Ann Plast Surg 2004;53(3):250–5.

24. Wong MZ, Wong CH, Tan BK, et al. Surgical anatomy of the medial sural artery perforator flap. J Reconstr Microsurg 2012;28(8):555–60.

25. Kao HK, Chang KP, Chen YA, et al. Anatomical basis and versatile application of the free medial sural artery perforator flap for head and neck reconstruction. Plast Reconstr Surg 2010;125(4):1135–45.

26. Lin CH, Hsieh YH, Lin CH. The Medial Sural Artery Perforator Flap in Lower Extremity Reconstruction. Clin Plast Surg 2021;48(2):249–57.

27. Lee CH, Chang NJT, Hsiao JC, et al. Extended Use of Chimeric Medial Sural Artery Perforator Flap for 3-Dimensional Defect Reconstruction. Ann Plast Surg 2019;82(1S Suppl 1):S86–94.

28. Chang NJ, Waughlock N, Kao D, et al. Efficient design of split anterolateral thigh flap in extremity reconstruction. Plast Reconstr Surg 2011;128(6): 1242–9.

29. Fu J, Gao J, Yi Y, et al. The Clinical Application of Medial Sural Vessels as Recipient Vessels in Repairing Traumatic Tissue Defects in the Lower Limbs. Ann Plast Surg 2020;84(4):418–24.

30. Dusseldorp JR, Pham QJ, Ngo Q, et al. Vascular anatomy of the medial sural artery perforator flap: a new classification system of intra-muscular branching patterns. J Plast Reconstr Aesthetic Surg 2014;67(9):1267–75.

31. Vanderhooft E. The frequency of and relationship between the palmaris longus and plantaris tendons. Am J Orthop (Belle Mead NJ) 1996;25(1):38–41.

32. Harvey FJ, Chu G, Harvey PM. Surgical availability of the plantaris tendon. J Hand Surg Am 1983; 8(3):243–7.

33. Alagoz MS, Uysal AC, Tuccar E, et al. Morphologic assessment of the tendon graft donor sites: palmaris longus, plantaris, tensor fascia lata. J Craniofac Surg 2008;19(1):246–50.

34. Zhao W, Li Z, Wu L, et al. Medial Sural Artery Perforator Flap Aided by Ultrasonic Perforator Localization for Reconstruction After Oral Carcinoma Resection. J Oral Maxillofac Surg 2016;74(5): 1063–71.

35. Abdelrahman M, Jumabhoy I, Qiu SS, et al. Perfusion dynamics of the medial sural artery perforator (MSAP) flap in lower extremity reconstruction using laser Doppler perfusion imaging (LDPI): a clinical study. J Plast Surg Hand Surg 2020;54(2):112–9.

36. Huang RW, Tsai TY, Hsieh YH, et al. Reliability of Postoperative Free Flap Monitoring with a Novel Prediction Model Based on Supervised Machine Learning. Plast Reconstr Surg 2023. https://doi.org/10.1097/PRS.0000000000010307. Online ahead of print.

37. Tee R, Jeng SF, Chen CC, et al. The medial sural artery perforator pedicled propeller flap for coverage of middle-third leg defects. J Plast Reconstr Aesthetic Surg 2019;72(12):1971–8.

38. Tsetsonis CH, Kaxira OS, Laoulakos DH, et al. The arterial communication between the gastrocnemius muscle heads: a fresh cadaveric study and clinical implications. Plast Reconstr Surg 2000;105(1):94–8.

39. Kao HK, Chang KP, Wei FC, et al. Comparison of the medial sural artery perforator flap with the radial forearm flap for head and neck reconstructions. Plast Reconstr Surg 2009;124(4):1125–32.

40. Wei FC, Mardini S. Freestyle free flaps. Plast Reconstr Surg 2004;114(4):910–6.

The Role of Microsurgery in Coverage of Defects of the Hand

Soumen Das De, MBBS, FRCS, MPH

KEYWORDS

- Hand defects • Complex injuries • Microsurgery • Surgical strategies

KEY POINTS

- The hand is a highly specialized region with specific reconstructive requirements.
- A large variety of nonmicrosurgical reconstructive options have been described for the hand.
- There are distinct situations where microsurgical reconstruction can provide better functional and cosmetic outcomes than conventional, nonmicrosurgical techniques.
- Radical debridement, rigid skeletal stabilization, and liberal use of free tissue transfer ensure that the extent of fibrosis after severe hand injuries is minimized.
- The pedicled groin flap still has a crucial role in the microsurgical era.

INTRODUCTION

Rapid advances in microsurgical technique, technology, and understanding of microvascular anatomy and physiology have made free tissue transfer relatively commonplace in our reconstructive armamentarium. The reconstructive ladder has been supplanted by the nimbler reconstructive elevator, which provides the surgeon with a more comprehensive strategy to address a particular problem. The main advantage of free tissue transfer is the flexibility it provides with respect to flap dimensions, composition, and pedicle length. Free flaps are often the first choice among many surgeons. However, are free flaps really "free"? Even though free tissue transfer has become technically easier, it still incurs significant time, manpower, logistics, and costs. We should be aware that the metaphorical elevator moves in both directions and nonmicrosurgical options work well in many reconstructive scenarios.

The aim of this article is to articulate the specific situations in hand reconstruction when microsurgery is superior to nonmicrosurgical reconstructive options. The benefits of microsurgical reconstruction include a variety of important metrics, such as improved function, better tissue match, less donor site morbidity, and reduced downtime for the patient.

RECONSTRUCTIVE REQUIREMENTS IN THE HAND

The hand is a highly specialized region, and it is divided into functional compartments. There is an outer soft tissue envelope, the underlying fibro-osseous framework, and the intervening "mobile unit" comprising the musculotendinous and neurovascular structures. In terms of reconstructive needs, the fingers require very thin and pliable skin that is tethered and well-padded volarly. The pulp tissue should ideally possess a high density of sensory receptors that provide an exquisite level of sensitivity and tactile discrimination to the fingers. On the dorsal surface, the skin is mobile, and the redundancy of tissue allows the fingers to curl up into full flexion while the specialized nail complex aids with fine prehension. The skin over the palmar surface of the hand comprises thick, non–hair-bearing glabrous skin, which is resistant to shear and pressure during grip. In contrast, the dorsal skin is thin, pliable, and has little subcutaneous

Department of Hand and Reconstructive Microsurgery, National University Health System, 1E Kent Ridge Road, Singapore 119228
E-mail address: soumendasde@gmail.com

Hand Clin 40 (2024) 221–228
https://doi.org/10.1016/j.hcl.2023.10.003

fat. It is pigmented, hair-bearing, and the more visible surface of the hand.[1] Because of these unique anatomic characteristics, primary repair such as replantation still provides better functional and cosmetic outcomes. When this is not possible, like-for-like reconstruction is the next best alternative (**Fig. 1**A and B). There are many other reconstructive options that have been described for the hand, ranging from skin grafts, a large variety of local and regional flaps, distant flaps, and free tissue transfer. There are many published algorithms for the management of hand soft tissue defects using local and regional flaps.[2] These approaches are popular because they are relatively easy, give reasonably good outcomes, and provide good exposure for trainees. However, they are not completely without problems.

PROBLEMS WITH NONMICROSURGICAL RECONSTRUCTIVE OPTIONS

Skin grafts are widely used for coverage of hand defects with a healthy bed. However, they inevitably lead to secondary contraction, provide poor volume replacement, and hamper subsequent procedures that may be required in the same field, such as tendon transfers and bone grafting.

Homodigital flaps such as the V-Y advancement, neurovascular island (NVI), and reverse vascular island flaps allow a single-stage reconstruction, and they do not damage another finger. However, they are only feasible in small digital defects because of the limited volume of tissue that is available.[3]

The cross-finger flap is a versatile *heterodigital flap* but it may result in significant stiffness in an adjacent normal finger and also results in a poor color match in patients with pigmented skin. It is very useful for fingertip defects involving the small and ring finger where an adjacent longer finger reduces the need for excessive finger flexion to achieve good flap inset. Other heterodigital flaps such the NVI flap from an adjacent finger cause scarring and loss of sensation in an unaffected digit and should be avoided if other options are available.

Regional flaps such as the posterior interosseous artery flap are useful because they limit the donor morbidity to the same limb and provide more tissue for larger defects. However, the distal reach of these flaps is limited by the location of the vascular pivot point, and they leave visible donor site scarring. The reverse radial forearm flap is a robust option but requires sacrifice of a major blood vessel to the hand. In contrast, perforator-based flaps such as the ulnar artery perforator flap preserve the main vessels but are only suitable for small hand defects with a narrow zone of injury.

The pedicled groin flap is an excellent *distant flap*; it can be elevated quickly, does not require microsurgical expertise, and a well-designed flap can allow the hand to be placed in a functional position.[4] However, it is still an inconvenience to the patient and requires multiple staged operations during a few weeks.

SPECIFIC INDICATIONS FOR MICROSURGICAL RECONSTRUCTION IN THE HAND

Considering the above issues, free tissue transfer provides some benefits that outweigh the costs and demand for resources. These include better

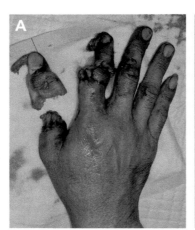
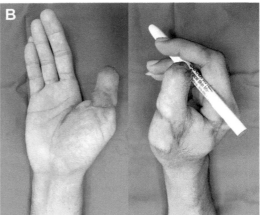

Fig. 1. (*A*) This patient had crush-avulsion injuries of the thumb and index finger. The tissues were extensively crushed, and replantation was not possible. Instead of performing a ray amputation of the index finger, the viable proximal phalangeal segment was transposed on to the thumb as a bipedicled flap (on-top plasty). (*B*) This provided length, a good web space, and an adequate sensibility to the thumb so that the patient could perform fine prehension tasks.

color, contour, and texture match, greater volume of available tissue, more concealed donor sites, and less functional downtime, both for the patient as well as individual joints. Of course, the surgeon must ultimately rationalize the cost-effectiveness balance with each case and select a treatment strategy that provides the best outcomes for the individual patient.

In this section, some important indications for microsurgical reconstruction in the hand are reviewed.

Large Hand Defects

The upper limb has a natural, tapering design with a larger amount of soft tissue in the arm and forearm and very less redundancy in the hand.[5] We have previously attempted to quantify defects in the digits and hand.[3,6] In the fingers, this can be done by considering the affected *surface* (palmar, dorsal, and combined) and *segment* (proximal, middle, and distal) of the finger. For the hand, a similar concept may be applied by dividing the hand into subunits. *Small-to-medium*-sized soft tissue defects can be covered with flaps from the fingers (eg, cross finger flap; NVI flap), hand (eg, dorsal metacarpal artery perforator flap), and forearm (eg, radial artery perforator flap). However, larger soft tissue defects demand a greater volume of tissue and inevitably lead to more donor site issues such as scarring and prominent contour defects. In these situations, free tissue transfer provides a larger volume of tissue while minimizing and/or concealing the donor site defect (**Figs. 2**A and B and **3**). The reconstruction can be performed in a single stage, and the patient can commence early mobilization to maximize joint motion and hand function. Subsequent procedures can then be undertaken on an elective basis to fine-tune the results, such as improving the appearance of the reconstructed area.[7]

An alternative to coverage of large defects is the pedicled groin flap. The specific indications for groin flaps are as follows: (1) extensive injuries where soft tissue is required to cover underlying vascular grafts, (2) situations with compromised vascularity, such as high-voltage electrical burns, (3) as a form of staged coverage prior to toe transfer, and (4) in very small children.[8] In these settings, free tissue transfer may not be feasible because of limited available resources, lack of suitable vessels for microvascular anastomosis, the need to preserve vessels for subsequent reconstruction, and small caliber of vessels, respectively.

Multiple Digit Injuries

Soft tissue defects involving multiple digits is a challenging scenario because large quantities of tissue are required, and there are often no suitable heterodigital reconstructive options available. Reconstruction in these situations requires a great deal of preoperative planning. More importantly, the surgeon must have a *clear reconstructive strategy* and be able to visualize the patient's treatment timeline well in advance. This is critical to achieving a good result. These patients also frequently require staged procedures.

The specific considerations for multifinger reconstruction include the following:

- Flap thickness

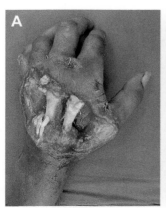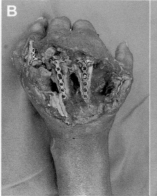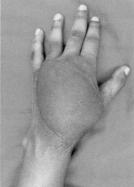

Fig. 2. (*A*) A large dorsal hand defect resulted from a crush injury, with multiple metacarpal fractures and disruption of the extensor tendons. At the initial debridement, all nonviable tissue including the interosseous muscles were removed and the fractures were temporarily stabilized with K-wires. (*B*) Rigid fixation was subsequently obtained with plates and screws and definitive soft tissue reconstruction was performed with a free anterolateral thigh (ALT) flap. The fingers and thumb were pinned in a functional position, allowing accurate templating of the flap and enabling healing with the tissues in their optimal resting state.

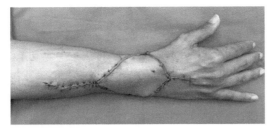

Fig. 3. A 57-year-old man presented with a large, fungating sarcoma originating from the dorsum of the wrist and forearm. After neo-adjuvant radiotherapy, a wide resection was performed, and immediate reconstruction was obtained using a free lateral arm flap. The flap has a similar color, contour, and texture as the adjacent area, and the microvascular anastomosis could be performed outside the irradiated area.

- Pedicle length
- Type of tissue

Finger reconstruction demands very thin flaps to permit finger motion. The surgeon must be aware that additional bulk is created when the flap is folded over for circumferential defects of the fingers and hand. Chen and colleagues summarized the thickness of commonly used flaps for coverage in the upper extremity.[9] Thin free flaps that are useful for soft tissue coverage in the hand include perforator-based flaps, fascia-only flaps, radial forearm flap (**Fig. 4**A and B), and lateral arm flap. An important recent advance is the pure skin perforator and superthin flaps that permit very thin tissue to be transferred using microsurgical technique.[10,11]

The flap pedicle length is an important consideration and depends on the zone of injury and the available recipient vessels.[12] Flaps with short pedicles include the pure-perforator-based flaps, such as the peroneal artery perforator flap. Axial-pedicled flaps such as the lateral arm flap have longer pedicles, approximately 3 to 4 cm. In situations where the microsurgical anastomosis must be performed further away, flaps with long pedicles are necessary. Examples include the medial sural artery perforator (MSAP) flap (**Fig. 5**A–C), radial forearm flap, and anterolateral thigh (ALT) flap. However, the conventional subfascial ALT flap is thick and secondary thinning procedures are required. An alternative to free tissue transfer is placing the fingers into abdominal or chest "pockets."

Some areas of the hand require specialized tissues, such as the palmar surface and the web spaces. The medial plantar flap[13] and superficial palmar branch of the radial artery[14] flaps are the only sources of glabrous skin besides the digits and may be used for the reconstruction of palmar defects of the hand. Del Pinal and colleagues have described free web space flaps from the foot to reconstruct web space defects in the hand.[15]

Critical Sensory Reconstruction

Restoring sensation is an important goal in hand reconstruction, particularly for soft tissue defects involving the thumb and index finger pulps that will affect fine prehension. A free toe pulp transfer allows the surgeon to provide like-for-like reconstruction with glabrous skin while simultaneously achieving sensory reconstruction and avoiding donor site morbidity in additional fingers[16] (**Fig. 6**A–C). Although not perfect, the final sensory recovery is acceptable and provides protective

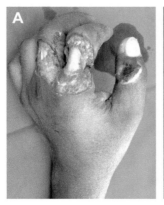
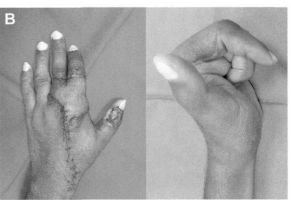

Fig. 4. (A) This manual worker had full-thickness burn injuries to multiple fingers, resulting in loss of the extensor mechanism and exposure of bone. Tendon reconstruction was performed using a palmaris longus graft and a free radial forearm flap (RFF) was used to cover the soft tissue defect. (B) The RFF is thin and provides a decent color match. The patient had good finger motion and declined further surgery to release the resultant incomplete syndactyly between the index and middle fingers.

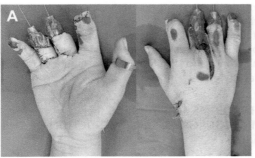
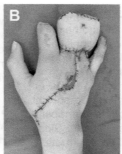
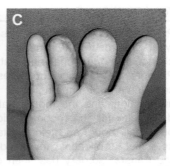

Fig. 5. (*A*) This 36-year-old man sustained crush-avulsion injuries of multiple fingers in an industrial accident. This resulted in circumferential defects of the middle and ring fingers, with loss of the distal phalanges. (*B*) A free MSAP flap was used to achieve immediate coverage. The drawbacks of this approach are that the fingers are initially bulky, an additional incision is required for the pedicle, and subsequent syndactyly release is required. An alternative is burying each of the digits in random-pattern chest or abdominal pockets and separating them a few weeks later. It is important to discuss the pros and cons of these options with the patient preoperatively. (*C*) The final appearance after separation of the webs and flap thinning is acceptable. Digit reconstruction with free toe transfers may now be considered to upgrade the prehensile function of the hand.

sensation.[17] I generally avoid free tissue transfer from the foot in patients with poorly controlled diabetes and peripheral vascular disease because of the higher risks of poor wound healing, infection, and potential digital loss from ischemia.

Composite Tissue Replacement

Composite tissue defects involve loss of skin, bone, joint, tendon, and neurovascular structures. There are 2 strategies for the reconstruction of these defects. First, the soft tissue defect may be covered with a flap, and nonvascularized grafts (tendons, bone, and nerve) can be used for the additional structures. The second strategy is using a composite tissue transfer, such as an osteocutaneous radial forearm flap and a tendo-adipofascial radial forearm flap.[18] The advantage of such chimeric flaps is that every component is vascularized, and healing occurs by primary intention, thus theoretically minimizing scar formation. Each tissue component is also in its native plane, and this is particularly important for tendon reconstruction. However, these flaps are technically very demanding because precise measurement and templating of each component is required so that the desired anatomic relationships can be achieved after the flap is inset. A poorly designed chimeric flap would require additional grafts, and this defeats the purpose of such a strategy.

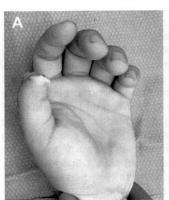
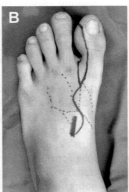
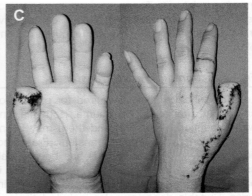

Fig. 6. (*A*) This patient sustained an amputation of the thumb with loss of pulp, bone, and part of the sterile matrix. (*B*) A free toe pulp transfer was performed. A long pedicle was used, and the microvascular anastomoses were performed to the dorsal branch of the radial artery and accompanying veins. The toenail was not taken because there was adequate sterile matrix left. (*C*) There is excellent color and texture match. In addition to providing like-for-like reconstruction using glabrous tissue, free toe pulp transfers simultaneously restore some degree of sensibility and do not require sacrificing sensation to another finger.

Total Digit Reconstruction

Partial and complete digit loss is another area where microsurgical expertise can significantly change the functional and esthetic outcomes. Patients may often elect to restore the normal complement of fingers rather than accept an amputation, and the foot remains an important donor site for the reconstruction of composite pulp, nail, bone, and joint digital defects. Since its initial application for hand reconstruction, toe transfer surgery has seen countless refinements and consistently provides good to excellent outcomes.[16] Wang and colleagues use a bespoke approach by taking elements of free tissue from both the great and second toe, augmenting intercalary segments with nonvascularized iliac crest bone graft, and assembling these to recreate a digit that closely resembles a finger in terms of length, girth, shape, and contour.[19] They also advocate using free tissue transfer to reconstruct the foot defect, thus minimizing donor site morbidity. Such procedures obviously require a high level of technical finesse as well as resources.

Vascularized Bone and Joint Transfer

In the hand, bone defects are seldom large enough to meet the size thresholds that have been commonly quoted for vascularized bone transfer. However, there are specific situations where free vascularized bone transfer may be considered in the hand. These include the following: osteoarticular and diaphyseal defects within a poor tissue bed,[20,21] interphalangeal joint reconstruction,[22] replacement of deficient carpal articulating surfaces,[23,24] and physeal reconstruction in the growing child.[25] These procedures produce reasonable results but prospective comparative trials are not available for such unique and complex scenarios.

Free Functioning Muscle Transfer

Loss of critical muscles required for prehension can occur after extensive trauma, ischemia, and wide resection of tumors, and there may be no suitable donors for tendon transfers. Free functioning muscle transfer (FFMT) has been widely used to restore finger, wrist, and elbow motion in paralytic conditions such as brachial plexus injuries. Suitable donor muscles include latissimus dorsi, gracilis, rectus femoris, and vastus lateralis, and the specific choice depends on the excursion, power, pedicle characteristics, and donor site considerations. The technique continues to be refined, and its use has been expanded to address

concomitant soft tissue defects and muscle loss with good outcomes[26] (**Fig. 7**A–C). Ongoing areas of research include minimally invasive approaches to muscle retrieval, donor nerve selection and matching, and longitudinal assessment of muscle viability.

STRATEGIES FOR SUCCESS IN MICROSURGICAL RECONSTRUCTION OF THE HAND

The severely injured hand is at high risk of fibrosis secondary to the persistence of nonviable tissue from marginal ischemia and unrecognized compartment syndrome, hematoma collection within dead spaces, unstable skeletal fixation, and infection.[27] The consequences of these are severe joint stiffness, impaired tendon gliding, and persistent pain from nerves that are transfixed in scar. The first step to minimizing fibrosis is radical debridement; having the option of free tissue transfer allows the surgeon to confidently remove all tissues of questionable viability. The role of microsurgery in the acute trauma setting is to revascularize the hand and digits with vein and/or arterial grafts.

The next consideration is to provide early vascularized tissue cover and a stable bony framework. Del Pinal and colleagues suggest that definitive reconstruction may be safely performed 24 to 48 hours after injury when there are adequate resources available.[27] A wide variety of free tissue transfers may be used to achieve coverage depending on the requirements—fasciocutaneous flaps for coverage of bone and implants, muscle flaps to eliminate dead space, and adipofascial flaps to maintain tendons in a healthy gliding plane. Early coverage must also be accompanied by rigid skeletal stabilization. This may be initially performed with K-wires (see **Fig. 2**A and B) followed by rigid fixation during definitive coverage. Negative pressure dressings are useful to seal off a well-debrided wound but prolonged use should be minimized because this leads to excessive granulation and obliteration of the adipofascial gliding planes. Having a brief delay between injury and definitive reconstruction is useful because it enables the surgeon to carefully formulate a treatment plan. During this time, additional imaging such as high-frequency ultrasound and computed tomography (CT) angiography should be obtained—these are invaluable in the selection and design of thin flaps, and this topic is discussed separately in this issue.

The most important benefit of microsurgery is that it facilitates early rehabilitation by greatly shortening the interval between definitive surgery

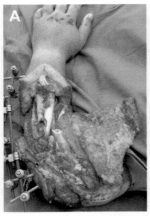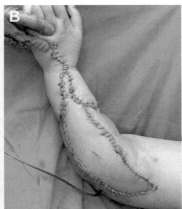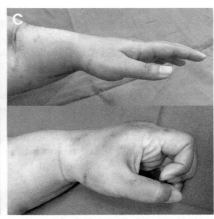

Fig. 7. (*A*) This patient had extensive forearm injuries with fracture of both bones and segmental loss of all the finger extensor tendons. After an initial thorough debridement, the fractures were fixed using plates and screws, the flexor tendons were repaired, and primary skin closure was possible. (*B*) A FFMT was subsequently performed with a myocutaneous gracilis flap to restore finger extension. (*C*) The FFMT allowed the patient to actively extend the fingers fully, and there was reasonable finger flexion to permit an adequate grasp. (Case courtesy of Dr Sandeep Sebastin, National University Hospital, Singapore.)

and rehabilitation. The defect should be templated in the position of function, with the metacarpophalangeal joints in flexion, interphalangeal joints extended, and the first web space fully abducted, so that the templated flap is of the correct dimensions. It may also be a good idea to maintain the joints in this position for a short period of time, either with splints or K-wires, so that the tissues heal in a functional position. Finally, the surgeon should anticipate secondary procedures, such as tendon and nerve transfers, improving the appearance of the hand and actively addressing complications such as joint stiffness and delayed union of fractures.

These strategies are likely to produce good functional results in a very challenging area of reconstructive surgery.

SUMMARY

The hand has unique reconstructive requirements, and a large variety of nonmicrosurgical reconstructive options have been described. However, there are distinct situations where microsurgical reconstruction can provide better functional and cosmetic outcomes than conventional, nonmicrosurgical techniques. The benefits of microsurgical reconstruction include improved function, better tissue match, less donor site morbidity, and reduced downtime for the patient. Mangling hand injuries are a prime example where radical debridement, strategic long-term planning, and versatile use of microsurgery can deliver superior clinical outcomes.

CLINICS CARE POINTS

- The hand is a highly specialized region with specific reconstructive requirements.
- A large variety of nonmicrosurgical reconstructive options have been described for the hand.
- There are distinct situations where microsurgical reconstruction can provide better functional and cosmetic outcomes than conventional, nonmicrosurgical techniques.
- Radical debridement, rigid skeletal stabilization, and liberal use of free tissue transfer ensure that the extent of fibrosis after severe hand injuries is minimized.
- The pedicled groin flap still has a crucial role in the microsurgical era.

DISCLOSURE

The author has no conflicts of interest to declare. No funding was received for this study.

REFERENCES

1. Rehim SA, Kowalski E, Chung KC. Enhancing aesthetic outcomes of soft-tissue coverage of the hand. Plast Reconstr Surg 2015;135(2):413e–28e.
2. Lemmon JA, Janis JE, Rohrich RJ. Soft-tissue injuries of the fingertip: methods of evaluation and

treatment. an algorithmic approach. Plast Reconstr Surg 2008;122(3). https://doi.org/10.1097/PRS.0b013e3181823be0.

3. Das DS, Sebastin SJ. Considerations in flap selection for soft tissue defects of the hand. Clin Plast Surg 2019;46(3):393–406.

4. Bajantri B, Latheef L, Sabapathy SR. Tips to orient pedicled groin flap for hand defects. Tech Hand Up Extrem Surg 2013;17(2):68–71.

5. Ono S, Sebastin SJ, Yazaki N, et al. Clinical applications of perforator-based propeller flaps in upper limb soft tissue reconstruction. J Hand Surg Am 2011;36(5):853–63.

6. Das DS, Sebastin SJ. Soft tissue coverage of the digits and hand. Hand Clin 2020;36(1):97–105.

7. Ng N, Das DS, Chong AKS. Secondary procedures after severe upper extremity injury. J hand Surg Asian-Pacific 2021;26(2):152–7.

8. Al-Qattan MM, Al-Qattan AM. Defining the indications of pedicled groin and abdominal flaps in hand reconstruction in the current microsurgery era. J Hand Surg Am 2016;41(9):917–27.

9. Chen HC, Tang YB, Mardini S, et al. Reconstruction of the hand and upper limb with free flaps based on musculocutaneous perforators. Microsurgery 2004;24(4):270–80.

10. Yamamoto T, Yamamoto N, Fuse Y, et al. Subdermal dissection for elevation of pure skin perforator flaps and superthin flaps: the dermis as a landmark for the most superficial dissection plane. Plast Reconstr Surg 2021;470–8. https://doi.org/10.1097/PRS.0000000000007689.

11. Narushima M, Yamasoba T, Iida T, et al. Pure skin perforator flaps: the anatomical vascularity of the superthin flap. Plast Reconstr Surg 2018;142(3):351E–60E.

12. Diaz-Abele J, Hayakawa T, Buchel E, et al. Anastomosis to the common and proper digital vessels in free flap soft tissue reconstruction of the hand. Microsurgery 2018;38(1):21–5.

13. Troisi L, Berner JE, West EV, et al. Medial plantar flap for hand reconstruction: a systematic literature review and its application for post-sarcoma excision. Ann Plast Surg 2019;82(3):337–43.

14. Mabvuure NT, Pinto-Lopes R, Iwuagwu FC, et al. A systematic review of outcomes following hand reconstruction using flaps from the superficial

palmar branch of the radial artery (SUPBRA) system. J Plast Reconstr Aesthetic Surg 2021;74(1):79–93.

15. Del Piñal F, Klausmeyer M, Moraleda E, et al. Foot web free flaps for single-stage reconstruction of hand webs. J Hand Surg Am 2015;40(6):1152–60.

16. Lam WL, Wei FC. Toe-to-hand transplantation. Clin Plast Surg 2011;38(4):551–9.

17. Lin CH, Lin Y Te, Sassu P, et al. Functional assessment of the reconstructed fingertips after free toe pulp transfer. Plast Reconstr Surg 2007;120(5):1315–21.

18. Adani R, Tarallo L, Caccese AF, et al. Microsurgical soft tissue and bone transfers in complex hand trauma. Clin Plast Surg 2014;41(3):361–83.

19. Wang ZT, Sun WH. Cosmetic reconstruction of the digits in the hand by composite tissue grafting. Clin Plast Surg 2014;41(3):407–27.

20. del Piñal F, Innocenti M. Evolving concepts in the management of the bone gap in the upper limb. long and small defects. J Plast Reconstr Aesthet Surg 2007;60(7):776–92.

21. Graham D, Sivakumar B, Piñal F del. Triangular vascularized free fibula flap for massive carpal reconstruction. J Hand Surg Am 2022;47(2):196.e1–6.

22. Lin Y Te, Kao DS, Wan DC, et al. Simultaneous reconstruction of extensor mechanism in the free transfer of vascularized proximal interphalangeal joint. Tech Hand Up Extrem Surg 2013;17(1):20–4.

23. Higgins JP, Giladi AM. Scaphoid nonunion vascularized bone grafting in 2021: is avascular necrosis the sole determinant? J Hand Surg Am 2021;46(9):801–6.e2.

24. Higgins JP, Bürger HK. Medial femoral trochlea osteochondral flap: applications for scaphoid and lunate reconstruction. Clin Plast Surg 2020;47(4):491–9.

25. Pho RWH, Patterson MH, Kour AK, et al. Free vascularised epiphyseal transplantation in upper extremity reconstruction. J Hand Surg Am 1988;13(4):440–7.

26. Fischer JP, Elliott RM, Kozin SH, et al. Free function muscle transfers for upper extremity reconstruction: a review of indications, techniques, and outcomes. J Hand Surg Am 2013;38(12):2485–90.

27. del Piñal F, Urrutia E, Klich M. Severe crush injury to the forearm and hand: the role of microsurgery. Clin Plast Surg 2017;44(2):233–55.

Microsurgical Treatment for Arteriovenous Malformations in the Hand

Mitsunaga Narushima, MD, PhD[a],*, Makoto Shiraishi, MD, PhD[b],
Chihena Hansini Banda, MD, PhD[c], Ryohei Ishiura, MD, PhD[d]

KEYWORDS

- Arteriovenous malformation • Flap planning • Classification • Pure skin perforator • Flap thinning

KEY POINTS

- Patients with arteriovenous malformation (AVM) of the hand should first be assessed for symptoms and staged according to the Schobinger classification.
- Ultrasonography and contrast-enhanced computed tomography are useful to confirm the extent of the AVM and the location of the arteriovenous shunt (nidus) to determine if complete resection is indicated.
- The use of a thin flap, such as a pure skin perforator flap, is recommended for flap reconstruction to minimize post-resection dysfunction.
- When pure skin perforator flaps are used, 2 veins are anastomosed to avoid the risk of postoperative venous stasis and venous thrombosis, and vasodilator medications are administered.

INTRODUCTION

The extremities are a common site of occurrence of vascular malformations, accounting for an estimated 60% of all vascular malformations.[1] Arteriovenous malformations (AVMs) of the fingers and hands are characterized by the presence of an arteriovenous shunt called a nidus that is usually located in the middle or tip of the finger which often prevents adequate arterial blood circulation to the fingertip. This causes poor blood flow, resulting in pain and ulceration of the fingertip. The prolonged blood flow insufficiency leads to atrophy of the distal phalanx and shortening of the digits.

Treatment Strategies for Arteriovenous Malformations

In addition to surgery, the following treatment methods are also used for AVMs: (1) embolization, (2) sclerotherapy, (3) drug therapy, and (4) laser therapy. Embolization alone using n-butyl-2-cyanoacrylate or isobutyl cyanoacrylate (IBCA) has been reported. There are reports of repeated IBCA embolization for pain control, but complications have been reported, including re-expansion,[2] neuropathy, skin necrosis, finger necrosis, and the development of collateral blood vessels after treatment.[3,4] In AVMs with major outflow vessels, coil embolization of the major outflow vessels followed by ethanol embolization of the nidus has been reported with excellent results.[5] Surgical resection is often followed by reconstruction of the resulting defect using flaps or skin grafts, as in cases where hand function cannot be preserved or distal necrosis may occur.[6–9] Following complete resection, no re-enlargement is seen, but the patient may lose a considerable part of the hand. Partial resection

[a] Department of Plastic and Reconstructive Surgery, Graduate School of Medicine, Mie University, 2-174, Edobashi, Tsu514-8507, Japan; [b] Department of Plastic and Reconstructive Surgery, Graduate School of Medicine, The University of Tokyo, Tokyo, Japan; [c] Plastic and Reconstructive Surgery Unit, Department of Surgery, The University Teaching Hospital, Lusaka, Zambia; [d] Department of Plastic and Reconstructive Surgery, Graduate School of Medicine, Mie University, Tsu, Japan
* Corresponding author.
E-mail addresses: sancho-ps@clin.medic.mie-u.ac.jp; sancho-ps@umin.ac.jp

Hand Clin 40 (2024) 229–236
https://doi.org/10.1016/j.hcl.2023.12.002

or ligation of the inflow vessel may result in re-enlargement, making radical cure difficult and causing acute exacerbation in some patients.[10,11]

Surgical Treatment of Arteriovenous Malformations of the Hand

The fundamental goal of surgical treatment is to achieve a complete cure by total resection to improve appearance, function, and relieve symptoms. However, because of its benign nature, aggressive surgical treatment may sacrifice normal tissue and function, and may even exacerbate the functional deficit. Furthermore, excisional surgery can lead to the worst-case scenario, including amputation of a finger and possible loss of life. These risks must always be fully discussed with the patient and his/her family to ensure they fully understand the risks, and informed consent must be obtained before the treatment is undertaken.

Timing of therapeutic intervention

In the case of AVMs, the Schöbinger classification (**Table 1**), a classification of clinical findings, is used for patient evaluation.[12] The timing of surgery is often reserved for stage III (pain, ulceration, bleeding, infection), where symptoms and dysfunction outweigh the risks of treatment, and the benefit outweighs the risk of surgery. However, the chronologic rate of growth must also be considered as it is sometimes better to proceed with treatment at a relatively early stage or when the disease is mild. This is particularly applicable when there is a trend toward enlargement at a young age, where the patient will likely reach stage III or higher, and when surgical treatment is deemed potentially curative. In elderly patients with little or no enlargement, observation may be a more suitable option.

Table 1	
The Schöbinger classification of arteriovenous malformations	
Stage	**Clinical Findings**
I. Quiescence	Warm, pink-blue, shunting on Doppler
II. Expansion	Enlargement, pulsation, thrill, bruit, tortuous veins
III. Destruction	Dystrophic skin changes, ulceration, bleeding, pain
IV. Decompensation	Cardiac failure

Adapted from Kohout MP, Hansen M, Pribaz JJ, Mulliken JB. Arteriovenous malformations of the head and neck: natural history and management. Plast Reconstr Surg. 1998 ;102(3):643-54.

How to determine the extent of resection

For AVMs, it is particularly important to resect the shunt portion with the nidus. Preoperative contrast computed tomography (CT) and angiography should be used to carefully confirm the location of the nidus. Cases with multiple niduses are not uncommon. In conjunction with the CT and angiography results, color Doppler ultrasonography may also be used to determine the entire area where the AVM is present and the extent of the planned resection.

For AVMs of the fingers, bilateral digital arteries and digital nerves are often resected at their bases. Regarding fingernails, if there is no obvious nidus in the nail matrix, the nail matrix and nail bed are best preserved from a cosmetic standpoint. However, excision of bilateral digital arteries may result in unstable blood flow, and normal nail growth may not occur. AVMs may also surround tendons. In such instances, the area between the tendon and bone is resected as much as possible. If necessary, the pulleys and ligaments are dissected and resected along with the AVMs. The distal phalanx is preserved, but the trabecular bone may be brittle due to long-term insufficiency of blood flow. This may eventually lead to finger shortening. Because of the many different variations in the vascular anatomy of the palmar region in AVMs, it is important to determine which branches from the palmar artery arch can be safely resected on CT to avoid postoperative finger necrosis. The dilated veins distal to the nidus are the result of increased blood flow due to the arteriovenous shunt, and we do not consider it necessary to remove all of them.

Necessity of preoperative embolization

Preoperative embolization is not often used in the hand. This is because the intraoperative blood loss can be controlled with the use of a tourniquet. Preoperative embolization carries the risk of anastomotic failure of free flap in cases requiring flap reconstruction. However, preoperative embolization may be used in cases where tourniquet placement is not feasible such as in upper arm AVMs. Here, preoperative embolization should be performed within 3 days prior to surgery because longer intervals allow for recanalization of the embolized vessel and development of collateral vessels.[13]

Method of Reconstruction

When primary closure is not possible, reconstruction is necessary for the fingers and hand. The ideal reconstructive modality should be well vascularized to cover the exposed tendons and neurovascular structures yet thin enough to maintain hand function, contour, and cosmesis. Reconstruction with a thin, flexible flap is recommended as skin grafts or thick flaps may cause postoperative finger or hand dysfunction. The superficial circumflex iliac artery perforator (SCIP) flap is the flap of choice, and it offers the added advantage of a donor site scar that can be closed primarily and easily concealed. However, the conventional SCIP flap is also too bulky to be used for the fingers, as despite the thin skin, the flap still contains considerable subcutaneous fat. Therefore, the authors recommend the use of a superficial circumflex iliac artery-pure skin perforator (SCIA-PSP) flap in which only the dermis and epidermis are used for the flap.[14] These flaps are also useful in cases of thumb defects and following toe-to-thumb and hemi-pulp flap transfers, for domino flap resurfacing of the donor site.

Thin superficial circumflex iliac artery perforator flap (superficial circumflex iliac artery-pure skin perforator flap)

The superficial or deep branches of the superficial circumflex iliac artery in the inguinal region are used as the vascular pedicle of the flap. Preoperative contrast-enhanced CT and color Doppler imaging should be used to confirm the anatomy and bifurcation of the branches. An incision is made in the inguinal region 1 cm below and parallel to the inguinal ligament, the vessels are identified, and the main trunk of the SCIA is confirmed on the central side. The superficial and deep branches of the SCIA merge 1 cm before the femoral artery and should be dissected carefully.

Three steps for pure skin perforator flap elevation

For PSP flap elevation, there are 3 useful techniques that greatly assist in the safe elevation of this flap.[15]

1. Primary thinning
2. Microdissection
3. Temporary clamping

Primary thinning: First, the flap is elevated, lateral to medial, at the level of the superficial fascial layer through a thin white film layer between the deep and superficial fat. Using this elevation method, primary debulking is performed with an electric knife without damage to the dermis or epidermis (see **Fig. 2**B).

Microdissection: Under the operating microscope, the flap vessels are confirmed. The pedicle and the blood flow are preserved during vessel separation from the surrounding tissues and dissection of extra subcutaneous fat. A branch of

the perforator is traced distally until it penetrates the dermis, this is the PSP. After detecting the position of the PSP, the path from the trunk to the position is marked on both skin surface and subcutaneous side to avoid inadvertent pedicle injury.

Temporary clamping: This is the last technique in PSP elevation method. After flap elevation at the superficial fascia layer, the main trunk of the pedicle vessels is temporarily clamped with a microvascular clamp. Temporary clamping is performed during this secondary debulking to prevent unwanted bleeding. Because a bloodless surgical field allows us to avoid unintentional injury of the PSP vessels and the dermal venous network, we can freely perform 3-dimensional defatting until the PSP flap is as thin as a skin graft (see **Fig. 3**B). After defatting is completed, the microvascular clamp is removed to reinitiate blood circulation in the PSP flap. Then, the pedicle vessel of the flap is dissected for transplantation. Through the application of primary thinning by elevation in the superficial layer, microdissection method, and temporary clamping, a PSP flap can be safely elevated and the thickness, folding, and final shape can be adjusted according to the reconstructive needs and the transfer completed.

Additional Surgical Considerations

The venous pressure in the AVM is often very high. Therefore, anastomosis of multiple veins from different venous systems is recommended to reduce the risk of flap necrosis due to venous thrombosis. If a superficial circumflex iliac vein is present, it should also be preserved and used for additional venous anastomosis.

In the inguinal region, vascularized iliac bone, sensory nerves, or sartorius muscle can be elevated at the same time and included as part of chimeric or composite SCIP-PSP flaps to replace like-for-like tissue removed due to the vascular malformation.[16]

Postoperative Care

Postoperatively, limb elevation of the affected limb is recommended along with intravenous prostaglandin E1 preparations (40 μg twice daily) and heparin 10,000 units/day, which are administered for 1 week. After the PSP flap, rehabilitation is started on the tenth postoperative day to prevent joint contracture of the fingers. Wire fixation of the fingers is not performed.

In the case of complete resection, recurrence is rarely seen, but recurrence from the surrounding area may be seen after long-term follow-up. However, there is no acute exacerbation from recurrence, and recurrence is often gradual and slight, so the patient should be monitored for follow-up.

Case

A 34-year-old woman presented with a pulsatile progressively enlarging swelling of the left little finger (**Fig. 1**A). She had mild pain of the finger. The fingertips were mildly painful and cold (stage III of Schöbinger classification). Preoperative CT angiography showed the presence of a nidus between the proximal interphalangeal joint and distal interphalangeal joint of the small finger. The digital artery on the ulnar side was identified with a tortuous course from the palmar arch, and the volar

digital artery on the radial side enlarged with a highly tortuous course distal to the bifurcation with the ring finger digital artery (see **Fig. 1**B).

After explaining the possibility of amputation, we planned complete resection of the AVM and SCIP-PSP free flap reconstruction. Preoperative color Doppler ultrasonography confirmed the presence of a large superficial branch of the SCIA and several branches.

Intraoperatively, the AVM was resected along with both digital arteries and digital nerves that were entrapped in the within. The dorsal cutaneous vein, which is the outflow tract from the nidus, was preserved.

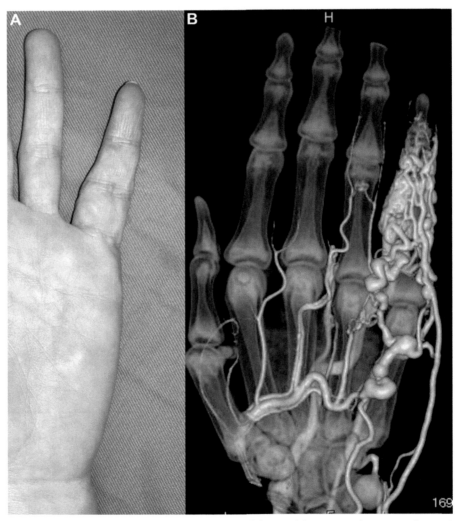

Fig. 1. (*A*) Arteriovenous malformations (AVMs) in left small finger. (*B*) Computed tomography angiography of AVM in left small finger. The AVM is present from the base of the metacarpophalangeal joint (MCPJ) of the small finger to the distal interphalangeal joint (DIPJ). The AVM of the ulnar digital artery is present from the superficial palmar artery arch and the radial digital artery is present from the common digital artery bifurcation. Nidus is present in the volar metacarpophalangeal region. The fingertips are slightly painful and cold. (Schobinger III).

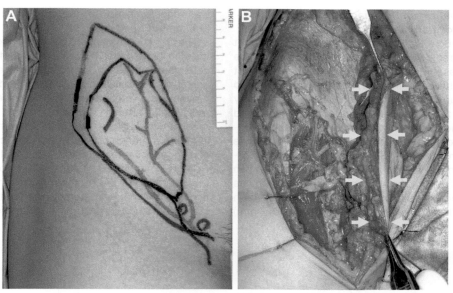

Fig. 2. (*A*) Superficial circumflex iliac artery perforator flap design on the left groin. The red line is a branch of the superficial circumflex iliac artery. The course of the vessel and its branches was confirmed preoperatively by echocardiography and marked. The purple circles in the groin are lymph nodes. (*B*) The superficial circumflex iliac artery was selected from the right inguinal region and elevated (primary thinning) in the superficial fascial layer. The thickness of the flap was about 1.5 cm, and a branch from the main trunk was followed peripherally under the microscope into the dermis (pure skin perforator) using microdissection. The *yellow arrow* represents the thickness of the SCIP flap before thinning.

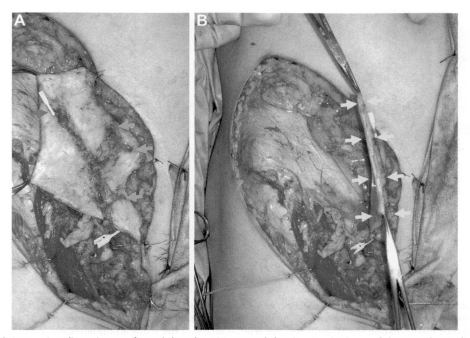

Fig. 3. (*A*) Once microdissection confirmed that the PSP entered the dermis, the base of the vascular pedicle of the flap was temporarily clamped and the surrounding fat layer was removed with scissors. The proximal side of the SCIA main trunk was clamped with a yellow clip to anastomose with the proximal end of the digital artery during flap transplantation. Green arrow: PSP, red arrow: peripheral end of SCIA. A slight fat layer was left on the skin flap to reconstruct the thin fat layer on the finger pulp. (*B*) Thickness of the SCIA-PSP skin flap viewed from the side. Yellow arrows show thickness of PSP flap. PSP, pure skin perforator; SCIA, superficial circumflex iliac artery.

Superficial circumflex iliac artery-pure skin perforator flap elevation and transplantation

An 11 × 6cm SCIP flap was designed in the right inguinal region with the superficial branch as the main vessel (**Fig. 2**A). The deep branch was not used in this case. Instead, the flap was harvested in the superficial fascial plane using the primary thinning technique as described earlier followed by microdissection and temporary vessel clamping to remove excess subcutaneous fat while preserving the 2 PSPs to complete the SCIP-PSP flap harvest (**Fig. 3**A, B). The main flap vessel, the superficial branch SCIA (2 mm), was anastomosed end-to-side to the palmar arch (2.2 mm) and the accompanying vein (0.5 mm) was anastomosed to the accompanying vein (0.7 mm). (**Fig. 4**C).

The fingertip was ischemic due to blood flow from the surrounding area (**Fig. 4**A, B). Therefore, it was considered necessary to reconstruct the anatomic digital arch circulation to improve perfusion and prevent cold intolerance.[17] To achieve this, the radial digital artery (1.0 mm) of the little finger was reconstructed using a vein graft (1.5 mm diameter) in-situ to a branch of the ulnar digital artery of the ring finger (1.5 mm diameter). The distal end of the SCIA (0.5 mm diameter) was then anastomosed to the ulnar side of the remnant digital artery at the fingertip (0.7 mm diameter) using the intravascular stenting method.[18] Lastly, the ulnar digital nerve

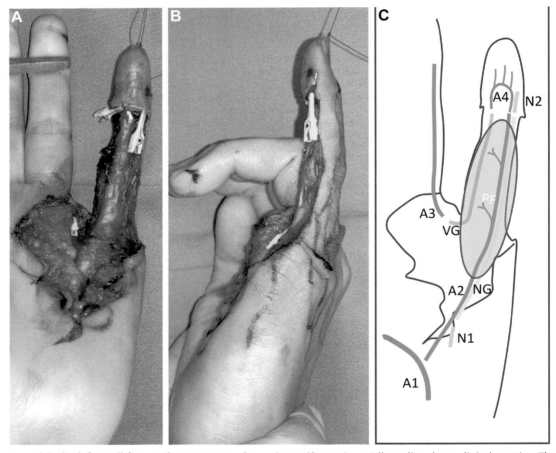

Fig. 4. (*A*) The left small finger after resection of vascular malformation. Yellow clips clamp digital arteries. The green clip clamps the vein. The fingertip of the little finger was poorly colored before resection of the remaining arteriovenous malformation (AVM) between the arterial arch and the metacarpophalangeal joint (MCPJ) of the ulnar finger artery. (*B*) Lateral view of the little finger after resection of AVM. (*C*) Schema of the reconstructive procedure. The proximal ulnar digital artery (A3) of the ring finger was transferred and the radial digital artery (A4) of the small finger was reconstructed with a vein graft (VG). The subcostal nerve was harvested from the right inguinal region and nerve graft (NG) was used to reconstruct the gap (between N1 and N2) of the ulnar digital nerve. SCIA-PSP flap was covered and anastomosed end-to-side to the palmar arch (A1 and A2) and further anastomosed end-to-end distally to the ulnar digital artery (A4).

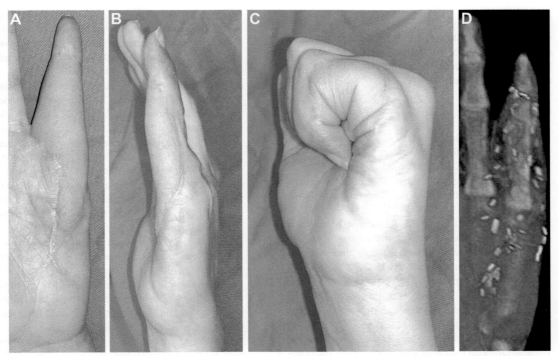

Fig. 5. (*A–C*) Twelve months after surgery. The flap was slightly thick, but no additional debulking was necessary. Full flexion and full extension range of motion of the small finger was possible. (*D*) Twelve months postoperative computed tomography showed no re-enlargement of the arteriovenous malformation (AVM) (numerous subcutaneous linear shadows are vascular ligature clips).

of the little finger was also reconstructed using a subcostal nerve (sensory nerve) included in the flap as a vascularized nerve graft and the wounds closed to complete the reconstruction (see **Fig. 4**C). The postoperative course was uneventful; the patient recovered well and was extremely satisfied with the functional and esthetic result (**Fig. 5**A–D).

SUMMARY

In the resection of AVMs of the extremity, a thin flap such as the SCIA-PSP flap, which is thin and flexible, should be used when flap reconstruction is necessary. There are various methods of thinning a flap. However, the flap can be elevated more safely if it is thinned using 3 key techniques: primary thinning, microdissection, and temporary clamping. When the venous pressure in the AVM is high, 2 veins from different venous systems should be anastomosed, and the affected limb should be elevated for 1 week.

In contrast to malignant diseases such as cancer, AVMs are not immediately fatal, but present the risk of losing an arm, finger, or even life due to heavy bleeding during treatment. For this reason, before performing surgery, the surgeon should fully explain the risks and ensure the patient and family understand the treatment plan.

CLINICS CARE POINTS

- Complete resection is the key to a complete cure in the treatment of AVMs.
- Preoperative CT angiography and Doppler ultrasonography should be performed to determine the extent of resection and the method of reconstruction. The attending physician should carefully consider whether the treatment is truly beneficial to the patient before treatment is performed.
- If venous stasis is suspected, 2 veins are anastomosed, and vasodilators are administered postoperatively.

ACKNOWLEDGMENTS

We are grateful to Dr Kohei Mitsui, Dr Kanako Danno, and Dr Kento Hosomi for helpful discussions.

DISCLOSURES

Conflict of interests: None. Statement of financial disclosure: None of the authors have a financial interest in the discussed article. No funding was received for this article.

REFERENCES

1. Mimura H, Akita S, Sasaki S. Japanese Clinical Practice Guidelines for Vascular Anomalies 2017. J Dermatol 2020;47(5):e138–83.

2. Widlus DM, Murray RR, White RI Jr, et al. Congenital arteriovenous malformations: tailored embolotherapy. Radiology 1988;169(2):511–6.

3. Hasegawa H, Takahashi A, Kamata M, et al. Treatment for arteriovenous malformation in a hand with transcatheter arterial embolization and surgical resection: a case report. Seikei Geka 2010;61(1): 41–4. in Japanese.

4. Park HS, Do YS, Park KB, et al. Ethanol embolotherapy of hand arteriovenous malformations. J Vasc Surg 2011;53(3):725–31.

5. Li X, Su L, Yang X, et al. Embolotherapy for high-flow arteriovenous malformations in the hands using absolute ethanol with coil-assisted dominant outflow vein occlusion. J Vasc Interv Radiol 2019;30(6): 813–21.

6. Hattori Y, Doi K, Kawakami F, et al. Extended wrap-around flap for thumb reconstruction following radical excision of a congenital arteriovenous fistula. J Hand Surg Br 1998;23(1):72–5.

7. Hibino N, Hamada Y, Aida Y, et al. A case of arteriovenous malformation (AVM) reconstructed from the wrist joint to the intrinsic finger area by arterial grafting. J JSRM 2005;18(1):78–82. in Japanese.

8. Watanabe T, Asato H, Umekawa K, et al. Resurfacing the index finger after resection of an arteriovenous malformation using a reverse forearm flap combined with additional venous anastomosis: A Case Report. JJSPRS 2012;32(5):335–9. in Japanese.

9. Guillet A, Connault J, Perrot P, et al. Early symptoms and long-term clinical outcomes of distal limb's cutaneous arterio-venous malformations: a retrospective multicentre study of 19 adult patients. J Eur Acad Dermatol Venereol 2016;30(1):36–40.

10. Sugioka T, Sunagawa T, Suzuki O, et al. Surgical Treatment for Arteriovenous Malformation Involving the Hand and Forearm. JJSSH 2008;24(6):940–3. in Japanese.

11. Furuya T, Nakazawa T. Congenital Arteriovenous Malformation of the Index Finger: A Case Report. J Jpn Coll Angiol 2009;49:430–3.

12. Enjolras O, Wassef M, Chapot R, et al. ISSVA classification. Color atlas of vascular tumors and vascular malformations. New York: Cambridge University Press; 2007. p. 1–11.

13. Mimura H, Akita S. Japanese clinical practice guidelines for vascular anomalies 2017. Jpn J Radiol 2020;38(4):287–342.

14. Narushima M, Iida T, Kaji N, et al. Superficial circumflex iliac artery pure skin perforator-based superthin flap for hand and finger reconstruction. J Plast Reconstr Aesthetic Surg 2016;69(6):827–34.

15. Narushima M, Yamasoba T, Koshima I, et al. Pure Skin Perforator Flaps: The Anatomical Vascularity of the Superthin Flap. Plast Reconstr Surg 2018; 142(3):351e–60e.

16. Narushima M, Hayashi A, Kaji N, et al. Surgical Treatment and Pathological Findings of Venous Malformations Involving a Nerve. J Reconstr Microsurg Open 2016;1:122–4.

17. Ishiura R, Shiraishi M, Narushima M, et al. Treatment of cold intolerance following finger pulp amputations: a case comparison between immediate finger replantation and delayed pulp and digital arterial arch reconstruction with flow-through free hypothenar flap. Case Reports Plast Surg Hand Surg 2021;9(1):33–6.

18. Narushima M, Mihara M, Koshima I, et al. Intravascular stenting (IVaS) method for fingertip replantation. Ann Plast Surg 2009;62(1):38–41.

Advances in Pediatric Toe Transfers

Xiao Fang Shen, MD[a],*, Saw Sian Khoo, MBChB[b]

KEYWORDS

- Toe transfer • Toe-to-hand • Pediatric • Microsurgery • Thumb reconstruction • Digital amputation
- Congenital hand differences

KEY POINTS

- Advancement in microsurgical techniques have expanded the indications for toe-to-hand transfer in both acquired and congenital hand defects to restore function, esthetics, and motion, with minimal morbidity to the donor site.
- Pediatric toe transfer demands high microsurgical skills and thoughtful planning due to the challenges and complexity of smaller structures compared to adults but the success rate is invariably high. Outcomes are generally good with the growth potential of the transferred toe and functional adaptation due to cortical plasticity in children.
- Microsurgical toe transfer techniques continue to evolve, and there is no one fixed method but a surgeon's versatility and innovation in using what one could spare within one's armamentarium because each case is unique.
- Esthetics and functionality are equally as important when considering hand reconstruction.

 Video content accompanies this article at http://www.hand.theclinics.com

INTRODUCTION

The innovative idea of toe-to-hand transfer was pioneered by Nicoladoni, in the nineteenth century.[1] He described the technique of staged second toe-to-thumb transfer, which required the hand and foot to be attached for several weeks. Buncke further developed one-stage microsurgical hallux-to-thumb transfer on 3 rhesus monkeys, with 2 successes.[2]

This was followed by successful one-stage microsurgical second toe-to-thumb transfer in adult by Yang[3] and great toe-to-thumb transfer by Cobbett[4] in the late 1960s. Ten years later, O'Brien reported the first pediatric toe-to-hand transfer for 2 5-year-olds with congenital absence of the thumbs.[5]

Since Nicoladoni, toe-to-hand transfer has seen an evolution from a staged procedure with prolonged immobilization, precarious blood supply, and less attention to nerve repair to a single-stage microsurgical reconstruction with emphasis on precise tendon and nerve repair.[3] Surgical techniques had initially focused mainly on ensuring the survival of the transplant, subsequently to reconstructing a more functional hand, and have now evolved to include attaining an esthetically "normal" hand while, at the same time, minimizing donor site morbidity.[6–21]

RECENT ADVANCES IN PEDIATRIC TOE TRANSFERS
Acquired Hand Defects

Microsurgical toe-to-hand transfer has become a good option in recent years for posttraumatic hand reconstruction in children with nonreplantable

[a] Department of Pediatric Orthopaedics, Children's Hospital of Soochow University, 92 Zhongnan Street, Suzhou Industrial Park, Suzhou, Jiangsu 215025, China; [b] National Orthopaedic Centre of Excellence for Research and Learning (NOCERAL), Department of Orthopaedic Surgery, Universiti Malaya, 50603 Lembah Pantai, Kuala Lumpur, Malaysia
* Corresponding author.
E-mail address: jane.78@163.com

Hand Clin 40 (2024) 237–248
https://doi.org/10.1016/j.hcl.2023.10.004

Table 1
Comparison of different types of free toe-to-hand transfer

Toe Transfer Techniques	Great Toe	Second Toe	Morrison wraparound[53]	Trimmed Great toe[8]	Combined Great and Second toe[16] (see Fig. 1)
Tissue harvested	Entire great toe (distal to metatarsal head)	Entire second toe (may include MTP joint and varying length of metatarsal shaft)	Entire great toe onychocutaneous flap with iliac crest bone graft	Entire great toe (medial part trimmed)	Partial great toe onychocutaneous flap with second toe osteotendinous flap
Number of joints possible	One	Three	None	One	Three
Appearance of reconstructed thumb/finger	Large and bulky	Small, bulbous tip, short nail, and tendency to claw	Good (but pulp instability common)	Good	Good
Appearance of donor foot	Obvious defect	Less obvious defect	5-digit foot	Obvious defect	Less obvious defect
Potential for thumb/finger growth	Yes	Yes	No (Bone graft resorption common)	Yes	Yes
Potential for great toe growth	No	N/A	Yes	No	Yes
Age suitability	Adult and pediatric	Adult and pediatric	Adult	Adult and pediatric	Adult and pediatric

amputation, failed replantation, and severe burn injuries of the hand.[22–24] Compared to other conventional methods such as distraction lengthening, osteoplastic reconstruction and pollicization, toe transfer elegantly restores length, stability, motion, sensibility, and esthetics while maintaining growth potential.[22] The level of amputation influences the selection of donor toe.

Full-length finger reconstruction

Various techniques for a full-length finger reconstruction have been described, each with its own set of limitations (**Table 1**). Great toe transfer gives better function and appearance than second toe transfer but results in more obvious defect in the

foot. A standard toe transfer cannot truly replace a finger, both in appearance and function, because both are not exactly alike. Since the introduction of a twisted-toe technique by Foucher[6] and subsequent variations in composite transplantation by Yu[7] and Tsai,[9] Chinese surgeons have described modified reconstruction techniques using free onychocutaneous tissue from the great toe to wrap around the osteotendinous components from the second toe to achieve a natural functional full finger reconstruction[11,12,16,19] (**Fig. 1**A-M). A customized reconstruction plan is templated from the measurements of the contralateral normal finger. Sun and colleagues transferred a great toenail flap together with part of

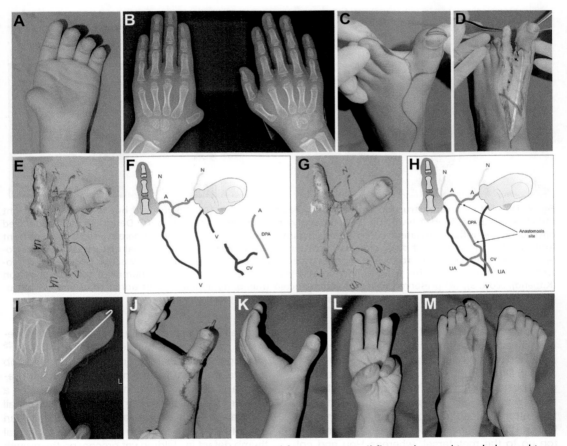

Fig. 1. Full-length thumb reconstruction with combined free great toenail flap and second toe phalangeal transfer. (*A*) A 6-year-old boy with congenital absence of left thumb. (*B*) Preoperative radiograph of both hands. (*C*) Operative design of donor site. (*D*) Arrow showing first dorsal metatarsal artery (FDMA), Gilbert type III. Deep dissection was not done. (*E*) The harvested great toenail flap and second toe phalanges with short FDMA pedicle. (*F*) Schematic diagram of (*E*). (*G*) Lengthening of FDMA pedicle with dorsalis pedis artery (DPA) graft and communicating vein (CV) branches. (*H*) The vascular anastomosis of FDMA to ulnar artery (UA) via DPA and CV graft. (*I*) The inset of great toenail flap and second toe phalanges with Kirschner wire. (*J*) Immediate postoperative appearance of the reconstructed thumb. (*K–M*) Follow-up at 3 months: (*K*) appearance of the thumb, (*L*) thumb opposition (Kapandji score 6), and (*M*) appearance of great toe donor site after resurfacing with second toenail skin flap.

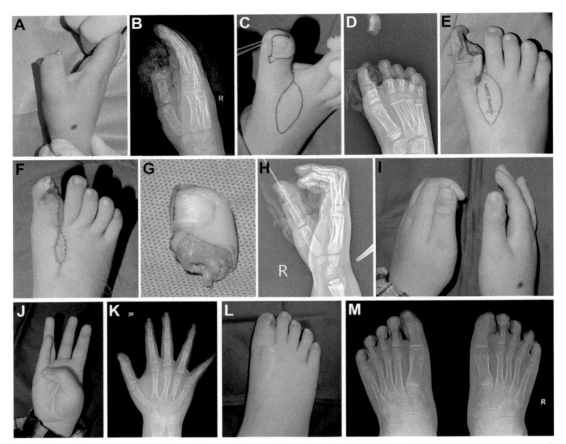

Fig. 2. Distal thumb reconstruction with partial great toe transfer. (*A*) A 5-year-old boy with traumatic right thumb amputation (Merle's level 1C). (*B*) Preoperative radiograph of the thumb. (*C*) Design of the vascularized onychocutaneous flap with lateral half of distal phalanx of right great toe. (*D*) Intraoperative radiograph of right foot showing the amount of distal phalanx harvested. (*E*) Donor site defect. (*F*) Dorsal metatarsal artery perforator propeller flap was used to cover donor site defect. (*G*) Great toe flap with short vascular pedicle. (*H*) Osteosynthesis with Kirschner wire. (*I–M*) Follow-up at 4 years: (*I*) appearance of the thumb, (*J*) thumb opposition (Kapandji score 9), (*K*) preserved physis of reconstructed thumb, (*L*) appearance of donor foot, and (*M*) radiograph showing growth and remodeling of distal phalanx of right foot to near-normal size.

the fibular distal phalanx to wrap around a vascularized second toe proximal interphalangeal (PIP) joint and used iliac bone graft in between to restore finger length and achieve the proper PIP joint positioning.[12] The second toe metatarsal head was retained to preserve the transverse foot arch. Instead of bone graft, Yin and colleagues[16] used the whole length of the second toe up to the metatarsal, whereas Hou and colleagues[19] used part of the great toe distal phalanx and both PIP and metatarsophalangeal (MTP) joints of the second toe for a full-length thumb reconstruction. The great toe donor site was resurfaced with the remaining second toenail skin flap.

Distal finger reconstruction

Nails are important ectodermal appendages that provide a protective and functional role including augmentation of precise touch, skilled hand movements, and ability to pick up tiny objects.[25] Although it is generally accepted that a thumb amputation distal to the interphalangeal joint retains an adequate functional level that negates a complex toe transfer surgery,[22] partial great toenail flap transfer with a short vascular pedicle[11,26] can beautifully restore the form and function of a distal thumb defect in children yet preserving the growth potential of the donor toe (**Figure 2A–M**).

Congenital Hand Differences

Toe transfer is commonly used for hand reconstruction in symbrachydactyly[27] (**Figure 3A–M**) and less commonly in constriction ring syndrome,[28,29] cleft hand,[30] macrodactyly,[31] and radial club hand.[32] Good functional and esthetic

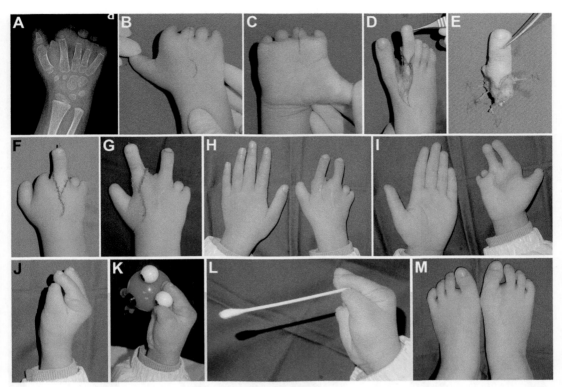

Fig. 3. Bilateral staged second toe transfers for basic hand reconstruction in type 3 monodactylous symbrachydactyly in a 4-year-old girl. (*A*) Preoperative radiograph of right hand. (*B, C*) Operative design. (*D*) Harvesting of right second toe. (*E*) Harvested second toe with short vascular pedicle. (*F*) Inset of toe to middle finger. (*G*) Vascularized left second toe transfer to index finger 10 months after first surgery. (*H–M*) Follow-up at 3 months: (*H, I*) dorsal and palmar appearance of both hands, (*J–L*) function of the reconstructed basic hand (Video 1), and (*M*) appearance of both feet.

outcomes can be achieved with toe transfer in congenital constriction ring syndrome[28,29] because the anatomic structures are normal proximal to the constriction site compared to that in symbrachydactyly or thumb hypoplasia. Nevertheless, achievement of basic hand function is still possible (Video 1). Unconventional donors such as polydactylous digits or functionless toes can be considered in cleft hand reconstruction when the usual donor sites are not available.[30]

Thumb hypoplasia

Anecdotally, toe transfer is controversial in modified Blauth type IIIB, IV, and V thumb hypoplasia. It is thought that the lack of a carpometacarpal (CMC) joint will result in a poor functional outcome after toe transfer, and pollicization is, therefore, the preferred treatment.[33] However, cultural differences and societal norms are strong considerations that are hard to ignore. In recent years, there has been an increasing interest in reconstructing unstable hypoplastic thumbs by means of toe transfers, in the quest to preserve a 5-digit

hand, with overall good outcomes reported comparable to that after pollicization.[14,15,17,18,34,35]

Luangjarmekorn and colleagues[35] described vascularized contralateral second toe MTP joint transfer to reconstruct type IV hypoplastic thumb. Ozlos and colleagues[34] also described second toe transfer with MTP joint arthrodesis, instead of tendon rebalancing,[36] to provide better stability and a longer metacarpal in the reconstructed thumb.

Instead of reconstructing the entire thumb, Tong and colleagues from Beijing Jishuitan Hospital preserved the distal thumb and used vascularized reversed second metatarsal to reconstruct the deficient metacarpal and CMC joint in type IIIB and IV thumbs, followed by other staged functional reconstructions.[15,18] This is also our preferred method of hypoplastic thumb reconstruction (**Figure 4**A–L).

The reversed metatarsal articulates with the trapezium, to mimic the CMC saddle joint, which is more natural than transferring the whole MTP hinge joint.[18] Vascularized second metatarsal is used in

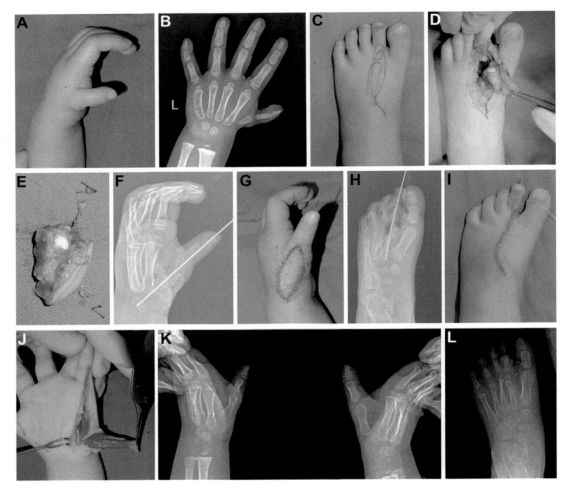

Fig. 4. Reversed vascularized second metatarsal flap for reconstruction of type IIIB thumb hypoplasia. (*A*) Hypoplastic thumb. (*B*) Preoperative radiograph of left hand. (*C*) Flap design. (*D*) Dissection and osteotomy of second metatarsal. (*E*) Osteomyocutaneous flap harvested. (*F*) The flap was placed in a reversed orientation, with the metatarsal head fixed proximally with a 0.8 mm Kirschner wire. (*G*) Wound closure. (*H*) Second metatarsal defect was reconstructed with partial longitudinal split of third metatarsal bone. (*I*) Donor site appearance. (*J*) Second stage abductor digiti minimi opponensplasty 6 months later. (*K, L*) Follow-up at 7 months: (*K*) Radiograph comparing both thumbs. (*L*) Radiograph showing growth and remodeling of donor metatarsals.

children aged older than 3 years while nonvascularized fourth metatarsal is used in children aged younger than 3 years.[18] Whole metatarsal transfer is more robust in size and shape compared to Chow's method of hemimetatarsal transfer.[10]

The common problem of soft tissue deficiency at the hypoplastic thumb can be addressed with an elliptical rotational flap from the dorsoradial wrist, thus reducing skin harvest and avoiding esthetically displeasing skin grafting at the donor foot.[17,18]

The donor toe does not need to be amputated; instead, the metatarsal defect can be reconstructed either by a nonvascularized longitudinal half-split or by a V-split of the adjacent metatarsal.[15,18] Both half-split metatarsals will eventually grow and remodel to weight-bearing width in children.[18] Besides routine opponensplasty, second stage surgery may include cosmetic lipofilling of the thenar eminence in selected patients.[18]

Good hand function (average pinch force of 1.5 kg in vascularized group and 0.9 kg in nonvascularized group, average Kapandji score of 6.7, grip and pen holding), radiological evidence of continuous bone growth, high parental satisfaction, and good donor site cosmesis and function have been reported.[15,17,18]

Refinements in Vascularized Toe Joint Transfer

Free vascularized toe joint transfers have been used to reconstruct a functionally important finger

---

Box 1
Author's preferred practice in microsurgical pediatric toe transfer

Surgical indications:

Absent/Deficient thumb with or without* CMC joint

Absent thumb and multiple fingers

Absent all fingers except thumb

Absent all 5 fingers (Metacarpal hand)

* *if parents strongly refused pollicization*

Timing of surgery: 5 years old

Preoperative planning:

Plain radiographs of the hands and feet

Digital subtraction angiography is not routinely done.

Preoperative preparation:

Preliminary cleansing of surgical sites with antiseptics day before surgery and fully covered with bandage to avoid contamination by finger sucking in children.

Intraoperative procedures:

General anesthesia with regional brachial plexus and popliteal sciatic nerve block

Urinary catheterization

Esmarch tourniquet at calf

Pneumatic tourniquet at upper arm

(Release every 1 h and rest for 10 min)

Microscope (minimum 20 × magnification)

Surgical techniques:

Donor choice for a full-length reconstruction: Great toenail flap wrapped around second toe osteotendinous flap

Approach to first toe web space: Distal to proximal dissection[54] **(Box 2)**

Donor site coverage: Local flap if small defect, artificial dermis (Pelnac, Gunze, Tokyo, Japan) if large defect

Method of bone fixation: Kirschner wire 0.6–0.8 mm

Vascular anastomosis: Prolene 10-0 (Ethicon, Johnson & Johnson, Puerto Rico, USA)

Nerve coaptation: Prolene 10-0 (Ethicon, Johnson & Johnson, Puerto Rico, USA)

Repair of ligaments and tendons: PDS 5-0 (Ethicon, Johnson & Johnson, Puerto Rico, USA)

Skin closure: Vicryl rapide 5-0 (Ethicon, Johnson & Johnson, Puerto Rico, USA)

Surgical time: 6–10 h (single surgeon)

Postoperative protocol:

Elevate hand and donor foot

Heat lamp for 7 d

Papaverine infusion 1.5 mg/kg, 6 hourly, for 7 d

Nerve block for vasodilatory effect and long-acting analgesia

No intraoperative or postoperative heparin use

Prevention of pressure ulcers

Intravenous fluid for 7 d

Antibiotics (cephalosporin) for 3 d

Immobilize both recipient hand and donor foot with cast (above elbow and above ankle)

Admission to general ward, accompanied by parents

No change in dressing for 1 mo and strictly no contact with water

Discharge after 7 d

Flap monitoring:

Serial clinical observation (Time-honored method)

Rehabilitation protocol:

Immobilize for 1 mo

Remove k wire in 1 mo

Start hand therapy after 1 mo

Allow full weight-bearing of donor foot after 1 mo

Compression garment for 3 mo

Secondary procedure:

Opponensplasty 6 mo later

---

joint in the growing child, usually due to compound defects from trauma or infection, with the aim to restore motion and retain its growing capacity.[37]

A recent systematic review reported that vascularized toe joint transfers have suboptimal range of motion and extensor lag deficit and highlighted some advances in reconstructive techniques.[38] Recent advances simplified the surgical technique and reduced morbidity from extensive dissection by transferring flaps on short vascular pedicles, with similar success rates.[37] Donor toes were not amputated as before but reconstructed with local flaps and joint fusion,[37] and some even recycled the resected finger PIP joint as nonvascularized bone graft for the donor toe.[38]

Box 2
Tips and Tricks: Author's approach in dealing with variable vascular anatomy of the foot

Tips and Tricks: Author's approach in dealing with variable vascular anatomy of the foot

- The arterial anatomy of the foot first intermetatarsal space is highly variable[55]
- Preoperative angiography may help but it is not routinely done
- Approach the first web space dorsally and dissect from distal-to-proximal as advocated by Wei[54]
- If the FDMA is dominant and superficial (Gilbert type 1), harvest the artery to the desired length
- If FDMA is deep, or first plantar metatarsal artery is dominant, do not proceed with deeper or plantar dissection. Instead, transect the plantar digital arteries at the bifurcation of the FDMA or just proximal to it (see **Fig. 1**)
- If both digital arteries of the recipient finger are favorable, direct anastomosis can be performed to the toe digital arteries
- A dorsalis pedis artery graft and communicating vein branches in the foot can be used to bridge the gap for conventional anastomosis to the radial or ulnar artery at the wrist (see **Fig. 1**).
- This method negates the need for deep dissection, which is more challenging, time consuming, and causes more morbidity to the donor site.

Lin described a novel technique to solve the extensor lag problem in vascularized second toe PIP joint transfer using the lateral bands, which is simpler than the Stack method of central slip reconstruction.[39] A reconstructive algorithm[40] based on the central slip of donor toe and extensor mechanism (lateral bands and lumbrical systems) of the recipient finger results in improved postoperative range of motion and reduced extensor lag.[38]

Nonvascularized Toe Transfer

Several authors have reported on successful nonvascularized toe joint or phalanx transfer in treating type III and IV hypoplastic thumbs.[20,21,41–43] Although it is widely acknowledged that nonvascularized transfer should be done before the age of 2 years old,[10,20,27] survival of nonvascularized graft in older children aged up to 11 years has been reported.[41–44] In our practice, the upper age limit for using nonvascularized toe transfer is

3 years old. Extraperiosteal dissection doubles the graft survival rate compared to subperiosteal dissection (90% vs 45%).[45]

Nevertheless, a recent systematic review of toe transfer for congenital hand differences showed that vascularized toe transfer has an overall higher success rate (98% vs 86.8%), lower resorption rate (0.7% vs 12.6%), less instability (0.7% vs 5.6%), and required fewer secondary procedures (19% vs 32%) compared with nonvascularized toe transfer.[45]

Reducing Donor Foot Morbidity

A systematic review found that donor site morbidity rates were much higher than commonly reported, with gait impairment in almost 24% of toe transfer.[46] Hallux valgus deformity was seen in almost 60% of patients with lesser toe transfer, and this was significantly correlated with foot fatigue, poorer walking, running, and other functional scores.[47] In contrast, most recent pediatric series reported no significant functional disability of the donor foot in the short-term, mid-term, and long-term follow-up of up to 13 years.[21,24,27,48] We postulate that children are probably innately better in adapting to such biomechanical changes in the foot compared with adults. However, we are unsure if such ramifications of toe transfer may be more pronounced in children as they grow, hence every effort should be taken in reconstructing donor sites whenever feasible.[15,20]

AUTHOR'S PREFERRED PRACTICE
Indications

We concur with Jones[49] that the considerations for hand reconstruction should be based on the actual anatomic deficit, rather than the etiologic deficit; but in addition, we included deficient thumb without CMC joint as an indication for toe transfer in parents who strongly refused pollicization (**Box 1**).

Surgical Timing

The optimal surgical timing is based on patient's size, comorbidities, and surgeon's comfort. Toe transfers should be performed early in life to allow better cortical integration and use of the new part in children but this must be balanced with the smaller structures, longer surgical time, and greater anesthetic risks in younger children. Although the optimal age is not known, the usual recommendation is between 2 and 3 years of age.[49] In our practice, we prefer to perform vascularized toe transfer at 5 years of age. The senior author has maintained a success rate of 100%, with no revision and no

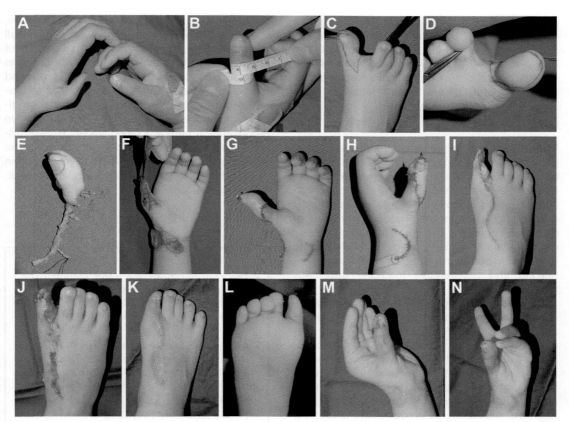

Fig. 5. Partial great toe transfer for congenital hypoplastic thumb. (*A*) A 5-year-old girl with hypoplastic left thumb and absence of nail. (*B*) Measure the contralateral thumb to determine the anticipated length, diameter, and nail size of the reconstructed thumb. (*C, D*) Operative design of donor site: (*C*) Dorsal view. (*D*) Plantar view. (*E*) Onychocutaneous flap with part of distal phalanx of great toe. (*F*) Preparation of recipient site. (*G, H*) Appearance of thumb immediately after transfer. (*I*) Donor site defect covered with artificial dermis, Pelnac (Gunze, Tokyo, Japan). (*J*) Appearance of donor site at 1 month follow-up. (*K–N*) Follow-up at 3 months: (*K*) dorsal view of left foot, (*L*) plantar view of left foot, (*M*) appearance of the thumb, and (*N*) Thumb opposition (Kapandji score 5).

requirement for postoperative intensive care unit admission to date with this age group.

Donor Foot Approach

The arterial anatomy of the foot first intermetatarsal space is highly variable. We describe our preferred method of approaching the donor foot in **Box 2**. Although this technique increases the number of anastomoses, it negates the need for deep or plantar dissection; hence, it saves time and reduces donor site morbidity (see **Figure 1A–M**).

Donor Site Coverage

As for donor site coverage, pedicles flaps from toes, feet or the lower leg, and free groin flaps have been described.[11] We avoid skin graft and prefer to use collagen-based artificial dermis, Pelnac (Gunze, Tokyo, Japan) because it is cosmetically pleasing and saves time (**Figure 5A–N**). It

can be used on exposed bone and tendon, and there is no need for subsequent skin grafting.[50] The dressing is removed after 1 month, followed by weekly dressing changes until the skin is fully epithelized, typically in another month.

Antithrombotic Agents

We do not routinely use antithrombotic agents intraoperatively or postoperatively. The usual cause of failure of toe transfer is due to poor surgical technique and inadequate postoperative immobilization. We think that antithrombotic agents alone do not play a significant role in maintaining the patency of microvascular structures.[51]

Flap Monitoring

Various methods have been proposed for flap monitoring following toe transfer, including pulse oximetry (pulse rate corresponds to arterial patency and oxygen saturation corresponds to venous patency),[24,33] laser Doppler, implantable Doppler probes, and indocyanine green with the SPY system.[52] We find the time-honored method of serial clinical observation of color, temperature, and capillary refill time sufficiently reliable.

DISCUSSION

With advancements in reconstructive microsurgery, the remarkable success rate of toe transfers has remained consistent in experienced hands. Hence, the paradigm should now shift to recreating not only a functional but also an esthetically pleasing hand and inconspicuous donor site that grows with the child. This is a major reconstructive challenge that truly marks the pinnacle of pediatric toe transfer, perhaps until the day that tissue engineering and regenerative medicine offer new hopes.

With the popularity of toe transfer as an alternative treatment option for thumb hypoplasia and increasing evidence of its good outcome,[14,15,17,18,20,21,34,35,42,43] we should probably reevaluate traditional teaching[33] and respect cultural preferences to preserve a 5-digit hand. In the modern world that uses more screen gadgets and technology devices compared with the past when manual labor was predominant, preserving an esthetically pleasing 5-digit hand at the small expense of a less-powerful thumb is an acceptable reconstructive option.[34] Surgical refinements are progressing, and longer term studies are much awaited to evaluate the true benefits of toe transfer in this group of children, perhaps at least until they reach skeletal maturity or enter the workforce. Only time will tell.

Outcome measures in current studies, if at all available, are mostly subjective and highly variable, perhaps because of the complexity of some congenital hand differences, lack of a normal contralateral side to compare in some, and difficulty in assessing young children. Nevertheless, a validated, objective measurement tool to standardize reporting of outcome measures is much needed to facilitate systematic evaluation of the outcomes of pediatric toe-to-hand transfer.

SUMMARY

Microsurgical toe transfer techniques continue to evolve, and there is no one fixed method. Rather, a surgeon's versatility and innovation in using what one can spare within one's armamentarium is essential because each case is unique. In recent years, there has been an increasing interest in reconstructing modified Blauth type IIIB, IV, and V hypoplastic thumbs by means of toe transfers, in the quest to preserve a 5-digit hand, with overall reported good outcomes comparable to that of pollicization. Toe transfers also see a surge in new surgical techniques preferring compound flaps using various combinations of onychocutaneous tissue from the great toe and osteotendinous components from the second toe to reconstruct a natural looking finger. Recent advances have also simplified the surgical technique and reduced morbidity from extensive dissection by transferring flaps on short vascular pedicles, with similar success rates.

CLINICS CARE POINTS

- The considerations for hand reconstruction should be based on the actual anatomic deficit rather than etiologic deficit with the primary aim of achieving basic hand function.[49]
- Anticipate variable anatomy (small or absent recipient artery) in congenital hand reconstructions and be prepared to anastomose to more proximal or unconventional recipient artery via grafts.
- Deficit secondary to trauma and constriction ring syndrome usually have normal proximal anatomic structures.[28,29]
- Deep plantar dissection to harvest a longer first dorsal metatarsal artery (FDMA) causes more morbidity to the donor foot. Flaps with short vascular pedicles have similar success rates.[37]
- The usual cause of failure of toe transfer is due to poor surgical technique and inadequate postoperative immobilization. Antithrombotic agents alone do not maintain the patency of microvascular structures.[51]

DISCLOSURE

The authors have nothing to disclose.

SUPPLEMENTARY DATA

Supplementary data related to this article can be found online at .https://doi.org/10.1016/j.hcl. 2023.10.004

REFERENCES

1. Carl N. Daumenplastik und organischer ersatz des fingerspitze (anticheiroplastik und daktyloplastik). Archiv für klinische Chirurgie. 1900;606.

2. Buncke HJ Jr, Buncke CM, Schulz WP. Immediate nicoladoni procedure in the rhesus monkey, or hallux-to-hand transplantation, utilising microminiature vascular anastomoses. Br J Plast Surg 1966; 19(4):332–7.

3. Yang DY, Gu YD. Thumb reconstruction utilizing second toe transplantation by microvascular anastomosis: report of 78 cases. Chin Med J (Engl) 1979; 92(5):295–309.

4. Cobbett JR. Free digital transfer. report of a case of transfer of a great toe to replace an amputated thumb. J Bone Joint Surg Br 1969;51(4):677–9.

5. O'Brien BM, Black MJ, Morrison WA, et al. Microvascular great toe transfer for congenital absence of the thumb. Hand 1978;10(2):113–24.

6. Foucher G, Merle M, Maneaud M, et al. Microsurgical free partial toe transfer in hand reconstruction: a report of 12 cases. Plast Reconstr Surg 1980; 65(5):616–27.

7. Yu ZJ, He HG. Thumb reconstruction with free big toe skin-nail flap and bones, joints, and tendons of the second toe–report of the cases. Chin Med J (Engl) 1985;98(12):863–7.

8. Wei FC, Chen HC, Chuang CC, et al. Reconstruction of the thumb with a trimmed-toe transfer technique. Plast Reconstr Surg 1988;82(3):506–15.

9. Tsai TM, Aziz W. Toe-to-thumb transfer: a new technique. Plast Reconstr Surg 1991;88(1):149–53.

10. Chow CS, Ho PC, Tse WL, et al. Reconstruction of hypoplastic thumb using hemi-longitudinal metatarsal transfer. J Hand Surg Eur Vol 2012;37(8): 738–44.

11. Wang ZT, Sun WH. Cosmetic reconstruction of the digits in the hand by composite tissue grafting. Clin Plast Surg 2014;41(3):407–27.

12. Sun W, Chen C, Wang Z, et al. Full-length finger reconstruction for proximal amputation with expanded wraparound great toe flap and vascularized second toe joint. Ann Plast Surg 2016;77(5):539–46.

13. Adani R, Woo SH. Microsurgical thumb repair and reconstruction. J Hand Surg Eur 2017;42(8):771–88.

14. Ozols D, Zariņš J, Pētersons A. Long-term evaluation of the functional and esthetical outcomes for the new method of the toe-to-hand transfer for full-length thumb reconstruction in congenital thumb's hypoplasia in children. Proc Latv Acad Sci Sect B Nat Exact Appl Sci 2019;73(2):171–6.

15. Tong DD, Wu LH, Li PC, et al. Reversed vascularized second metatarsal flap for reconstruction of Manske type IIIB and IV thumb hypoplasia with reduced donor site morbidity. Chin Med J (Engl) 2019; 132(21):2565–71.

16. Yin Y, Tao X, Li Y, et al. Cosmetic and functional results of a newly reconstructed thumb by combining the phalanx of second toe and the great toenail flap transplantation. J Orthop Surg Res 2020;15(1): 458.

17. Liu B, Chen S, Chow ECS, et al. Type IIIB and IV hypoplastic thumb reconstruction with non-vascularized fourth metatarsal. J Hand Surg Eur Vol 2020;45(7): 722–8.

18. Liu B, Bai F, Chen S. Revisiting the management of Manske Type 3B and 4 thumb hypoplasia. J Hand Surg Eur Vol 2021;46(1):21–9.

19. Hou C, Zhang A, Yu X, et al. Reconstruction of fully shaped fingers using a free great toe nail flap combined with a second toe tissue flap. Int Wound J 2022;19(6):1389–96.

20. Zargarbashi R, Panjavi B, Bozorgmanesh M. Congenital hypoplastic thumbs treated by staged nonvascularized MTP joint transfer for absent MCP joints and abductor digiti minimi tendon transfer for opposition: a case series study. BMC Musculoskelet Disord 2023;24(1):179.

21. Chughtai M, McConaghy K, Bui X, et al. Surgical technique and outcomes of reconstruction for blauth type III thumb hypoplasia. Hand (N Y) 2023;18(3): 413–20.

22. Jones NF, Clune JE. Thumb amputations in children: classification and reconstruction by microsurgical toe transfers. J Hand Surg Am 2019;44(6):e519.

23. Jones NF, Graham D, Au K. Bilateral metacarpal hands: reconstruction with 6 toe transfers. Hand (N Y) 2020;15(4):465–71.

24. Yoon AP, Jones NF. Long-Term outcomes after toe-to-thumb transfers for burn reconstruction in children. J Burn Care Res 2022;43(2):440–4.

25. Zook EG. Anatomy and physiology of the perionychium. Clin Anat 2003;16(1):1–8.

26. Hirase Y, Kanno Y, Okubo A, et al. Distal finger reconstruction technique combining a distally-based finger flap and a partial toe flap. Microsurgery 2023;43(3):222–8.

27. Sabapathy SR, Mohan M, Shanmugakrishnan RR. Nonvascularized free toe phalangeal transfers in congenital hand differences: radiological, functional, and patient/parent-reported outcomes. J Hand Surg Am 2021;46(12):1124 e1–e1124 e9.

28. Wang P, Jones NF. Salvage reconstruction of a congenital hypoplastic thumb due to constriction ring syndrome using a third toe transfer, when the usual donor sites of index finger, great and second toes are not available. HAND 2022;17(1):NP1–4.

29. Chiu DTW, Patel A, Sakamoto S, et al. The impact of microsurgery on congenital hand anomalies associated with amniotic band syndrome. Plast Reconstr Surg Glob Open 2018;6(4):e1657.

30. Taghinia AH, Taylor EM, Winograd J, et al. Digital transfer for hand reconstruction in cleft hand and foot differences. J Reconstr Microsurg 2021;37(7): 589–96.

31. Cavadas PC, Thione A. Treatment of Hand Macrodactyly With Resection and Toe Transfers. J Hand Surg Am 2018;43(4):388 e1–e388 e6.

32. Vilkki SK, Paavilainen P. Vascularized second metatarsophalangeal joint transfer for radial deficiency - an update. J Hand Surg Eur Vol 2018;43(9):907–18.

33. Jones NF. Toe-to-hand transfers in children. In: Abzug JM, Kozin SH, Zlotolow DA, editors. The pediatric upper extremity. New York: Springer; 2015. p. 483–511.

34. Ozols D, Butnere MM, Petersons A. The second toe-to-hand transfer for full-length thumb reconstruction in congenital thumb's grade IIIb to V hypoplasia: MTPJ arthrodesis instead of tendon rebalansing. Tech Hand Up Extrem Surg 2020;24(1):13–9.

35. Luangjarmekorn P, Pongernnak N, Kitidumrongsook P. Vascularized toe joint transfer for hypoplastic thumb type IV. Tech Hand Up Extrem Surg 2021;25(4):226–34.

36. Tu YK, Yeh WL, Sananpanich K, et al. Microsurgical second toe-metatarsal bone transfer for reconstructing congenital radial deficiency with hypoplastic thumb. J Reconstr Microsurg 2004;20(3):215–25.

37. Dautel G. Vascularized toe joint transfers to the hand for PIP or MCP reconstruction. Hand Surg Rehabil 2018;37(6):329–36.

38. Zhou KJ, Graham DJ, Lawson RD, et al. Toe-to-finger vascularized joint transfers for proximal interphalangeal joint reconstruction: a systematic review. Hand (N Y) 2022;17(6):1031–8.

39. Lin YT, Loh CY. A novel technique for correcting extensor lag in vascularized toe PIP joint transfers. Tech Hand Up Extrem Surg 2016;20(3):104–7.

40. Loh CYY, Hsu CC, Lin CH, et al. Customizing extensor reconstruction in vascularized toe joint transfers to finger proximal interphalangeal joints: a strategic approach for correcting extensor lag. Plast Reconstr Surg 2017;139(4):915–22.

41. Nakada M, Tada K, Nakajima T, et al. A case of a 5-year-old boy with a blauth type IIIB hypoplastic thumb reconstructed with a nonvascularized, hemi-longitudinal metatarsal transfer. Case Rep Orthop 2018;2018:8205285.

42. Kawabata H, Tamura D, Goldfarb CA. Treatment of blauth type IIIB thumb hypoplasia using a nonvascularized toe phalanx. J Hand Surg Am 2021; 46(1):68 e1–e68 e7.

43. Balakrishnan G, Vijayaragavan S, Somesh B. Restoration of five digit hand in type III B & C thumb hypoplasia-a game changer in surgical management. Indian J Plast Surg 2020;53(3):349–56.

44. Trost JG, Kaufman M, Netscher DT. Nonvascularized toe joint transfers to the hand in young children: technique revisited. Hand (N Y) 2022;17(4):676–83.

45. Meyers A, Bassiri Gharb B, Rampazzo A. A systematic review of vascularized and nonvascularized toe transfer for reconstruction of congenital hand differences. Plast Reconstr Surg 2023;151(6): 1256–73.

46. Sosin M, Lin CH, Steinberg J, et al. Functional donor site morbidity after vascularized toe transfer procedures: a review of the literature and biomechanical consideration for surgical site selection. Ann Plast Surg 2016;76(6):735–42.

47. Kotkansalo T, Elo P, Luukkaala T, et al. Long-term effects of toe transfers on the donor feet. J Hand Surg Eur Vol 2014;39(9):966–76.

48. Raizman NM, Reid JA, Meisel AF, et al. Long-term donor-site morbidity after free, nonvascularized toe phalanx transfer for congenital differences of the hand. J Hand Surg Am 2020;45(2):154 e1–e154 e7.

49. Jones NF, Kaplan J. Indications for microsurgical reconstruction of congenital hand anomalies by toe-to-hand transfers. Hand (N Y) 2013;8(4):367–74.

50. Lou X, Xue H, Li G, et al. One-stage pelnac reconstruction in full-thickness skin defects with bone or tendon exposure. Plast Reconstr Surg Glob Open 2018;6(3):e1709.

51. Veravuthipakorn L, Veravuthipakorn A. Microsurgical free flap and replantation without antithrombotic agents. J Med Assoc Thai 2004;87(6):665–9.

52. Levin LS. From replantation to transplantation: the evolution of orthoplastic extremity reconstruction. J Orthop Res 2022. https://doi.org/10.1002/jor. 25488.

53. Morrison WA, O'Brien BM, MacLeod AM. Thumb reconstruction with a free neurovascular wrap-around flap from the big toe. J Hand Surg Am 1980;5(6):575–83.

54. Wei FC, Silverman RT, Hsu WM. Retrograde dissection of the vascular pedicle in toe harvest. Plast Reconstr Surg 1995;96(5):1211–4.

55. Hou Z, Zou J, Wang Z, et al. Anatomical classification of the first dorsal metatarsal artery and its clinical application. Plast Reconstr Surg 2013;132(6): 1028e–39e.

The Foot as a Donor Site for Reconstruction in the Hand

Jorge G. Boretto, MD*, Fernando Holc, MD,
Pedro Bronenberg Victorica, MD

KEYWORDS

• Toe transfer • Great toe transfer • Microsurgical reconstruction • Hand reconstruction

KEY POINTS

- The dorsalis pedis-first dorsal metatarsal artery system provides different types of tissue, which can be harvested or isolated as compound or chimeric flaps.
- The versatility of the great toe transfer has allowed for reconstruction of not only the thumb distal to the metacarpophalangeal joint but also the fingertip.
- The twisted-toe technique and its modifications permit reconstructing a thumb with an amputation proximal to the metacarpophalangeal joint.
- The second and third toe transfers are useful for reconstructing single or multiple fingers, with cosmetic and functional outcomes dependent on a number of preoperative factors.
- Custom-made reconstruction of the thumb and fingers can be achieved by means of onycho-osteo-cutaneous, vascularized bone, or vascularized joint transfers.

INTRODUCTION

A special repository of tissues for hand reconstruction can be found in the foot. Over the last decades, numerous reconstructive options have been presented and embraced, including modifications of previously described techniques or even new options in hand reconstruction. In addition, foot tissue can be transplanted to reconstruct missing fingers or other hand tissues, rather than sacrificing viable tissue from an already injured hand.

Although Cobbett[1] is usually mentioned as the first surgeon to perform a successful great toe-to-thumb transfer in 1969 after the experimental work of Harry Buncke and colleagues,[2] surgeons in China performed the first microvascular toe-to-thumb transfer in 1965.[3] As a result, the foot has become a crucial site for hand reconstructive donors in cases not only of thumb and finger reconstruction but also for the hand. Most of the tissues transferred to the hand from the foot arise from the dorsalis pedis artery (DPA)-first dorsal metatarsal artery (FDMA) system.

In this article, we review the anatomy of the DPA-FDMA system and the flaps that have been described in this angiosome.[4] Our primary focus will be on surgical procedures that have been shown to be effective in the reconstruction of composite hand defects.

VASCULAR ANATOMY OF THE DORSALIS PEDIS-FIRST DORSAL METATARSAL ARTERY SYSTEM

Dorsalis Pedis Artery

The DPA is the terminal branch of the anterior tibial artery and originates anterior to the ankle joint,

Hand and Upper Extremity Surgery Department, Prof. Dr. "Carlos Ottolenghi Institute", Hospital Italiano de Buenos Aires
* Corresponding author. Hand and Upper Extremity Surgery Department, Prof. Dr. "Carlos Ottolenghi Institute", Hospital Italiano de Buenos Aires, Tte. Gral. J.D. Perón 4190, Ciudad Autónoma de Buenos Aires C1198AAW, Argentina.
E-mail address: jorge.boretto@hospitalitaliano.org.ar

Hand Clin 40 (2024) 249–258
https://doi.org/10.1016/j.hcl.2023.08.009
0749-0712/24/© 2023 Elsevier Inc. All rights reserved.

halfway between the malleoli. At the extensor retinaculum, it passes beneath the extensor hallucis longus tendon before descending as the deep plantar artery between the heads of the first dorsal interosseous muscle to meet the lateral plantar branch of the posterior tibial artery at the plantar arch in the sole of the foot. The medial and lateral tarsal arteries, the arcuate artery, the FDMA, and cutaneous branches to the medial side of the foot are the DPAs branches. Several anatomic and in vivo studies have shown that the dorsal foot arterial distribution is highly variable.[5–7] The dorsalis pedis origin can be the peroneal artery, or it can be slender or absent between 5.7%[8] and 9.4%.[5] In these later cases, the FDMA was derived from the lateral metatarsal artery instead of the DPA.[5]

The terminal branch of the DPA is the FDMA, which has been more extensively studied because it gives the origin of the vessels for the first and second toes. All the authors report variability in the course of the FDMA, with some differences.[5,7–10] Gilbert classified the vessels in the first metatarsal space based on the anatomy of the first web space and its relationship to the first dorsal interosseous muscle. The FDMA was classified into three different types.[11] In the majority of specimens, the artery was superficial or lay on the surface of the muscle, consistent with type 1. In type 2, the location of the artery was deep within the muscle. In type 3, the dorsal arteries were extremely thin, and the first plantar metatarsal artery (FPMA) supplied the vascularization. Leung and Wong[8] classified the FDMA according to the depth in the first metatarsal space into seven types. This classification overlaps with Gilberts' classification. May and colleagues[12] and Lee and Dauber[5] simplified the classification by dividing the origin of the FDMA into superficial or deep. Moreover, May and colleagues[12] described three patterns of the distal communicating artery (DCA) between the dorsal and plantar metatarsal arteries. Spanio and colleagues[13] examined the DCA, and the diameters of the FDMA, and FPMA to determine whether the vascular dominance was dorsal or plantar and how symmetric it was in patients who had both second toes transferred. They found that 78% of patients had symmetric anatomy of the vascular pedicle, with 62% dorsal artery dominance and 16% plantar artery dominance. Based on an anatomic study of 148 patients and 48 cadaveric dissections, Hou and colleagues[10] described the ABC (**A**rise, **B**ranch, and **C**ourse) classification for the FDMA. In contrast to Gilbert's classification, they do not find an intramuscular pattern in the FDMA. Instead, they say that 84% of the time, the FDMA runs

between the first metatarsal and the first dorsal intermetatarsal muscle.

FLAPS FROM THE DORSALIS PEDIS ARTERY
Dorsalis Pedis Flap

The dorsalis pedis flap was first described by McCRaw and Furlow.[14] It quickly became popular due to its flexibility, nerve supply, and thickness, especially in hand reconstruction, where bulky flaps should be avoided (**Fig. 1**). The main concern regarding the use of the dorsalis pedis has been donor-site morbidity,[15] although some proponents have attributed complications at the donor site to technical factors.[16] The development of perforator flaps has primarily limited their use as a result of these disadvantages.[17] However, the dorsalis pedis flap as a composite or chimeric flap has shown itself to be useful in compound defects of the hand.[18–20] Chung and Tong[18] reported a case of a compound free dorsalis pedis flap along with the great toe trimmed flap and the second toe fillet flap. Although reported as a conjoint flap, this reconstruction corresponds to a chimeric flap in the updated simplified nomenclature for compound flaps.[20] Xie and colleagues[21] described the use of a chimeric dorsalis pedis flap to reconstruct the dorsum of multiple fingers in two cases. In both cases, they harvested three flaps based on the dorsalis pedis and its branches, namely, the medial and lateral tarsal arteries. This approach allowed a single-stage reconstruction in the case of a three finger dorsal coverage defect.

When the extensor tendons of the hand have been lost and the dorsal defect of the hand needs to be covered, the dorsalis pedis tendinocutaneous flap can be used to do a completely vascularized, one-stage reconstruction with the dorsalis pedis tendinocutaneous flap.[22] In these cases, the skin flap is elevated along with the extensor digitorum longus tendons. The advantages of vascularized tendons are faster healing and lesser adhesion formation, enabling unrestricted gliding.[23–25] Lee and colleagues performed this reconstruction in 13 patients with combined tendinocutaneous defects of the hand and wrist.[24] As a complication at the recipient site, two patients had tendon adhesions and underwent tenolysis. On the contrary, at the donor site, there were no immediate postoperative complications. However, at long-term follow-up, there was skin breakdown in one case and scar contracture in another patient.

Adani and colleagues[23] reported the results on seven patients with tendinocutaneous defects of the dorsal hand with this approach. At a minimum follow-up of 28 months, the investigators reported that there were no tendon adhesions and the

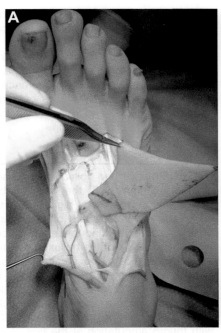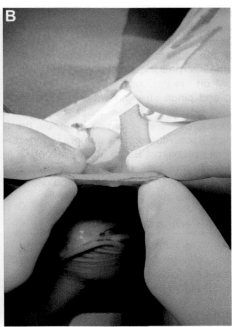

Fig. 1. (*A*) The dorsalis pedis flap is harvested from the foot with the dorsalis pedis artery (*red vessel loop*), the great saphenous vein (*blue vessel loop*), and the superficial peroneal nerve. (*B*) Thickness of the dorsalis pedis flap.

tendons functioned well, but no range of motion (ROM) was described. However, six out of seven patients had donor site complications with partial skin graft loss. The investigators mentioned that, even with the complications at the donor site, the benefits of the procedure outweighed the donor-site morbidity.

Extensor Digitorum Brevis Flap

The lateral tarsal artery, a branch of the DPA, provides the arterial supply for the extensor digitorum brevis (EDB) muscle.[26] This flap has been used as a composite flap or as a chimeric flap in hand reconstruction.[26–30] Interestingly, the EDB muscle flap has been used as a free functional muscle transfer to reconstruct the adductor pollicis muscle[28] and the opponens pollicis muscle.[29,30] All the reported cases achieved reinnervation and enough strength to perform the planned mobility.

The EDB flap has also been described as a flow-through flap.[26] However, it should be noted that the coverage capabilities of the flap are small (20 cm^2 on average), and for more extended coverage defects, a dorsalis pedis adipofascial-EDB-free chimeric flap can be used.[26]

FLAPS FROM THE FIRST METATARSAL ARTERIES

The first metatarsal artery, either dorsal or plantar dominant, provides the vascular supply for the

great toe and second toe, among other tissues. Since the first report of a great toe transfer to reconstruct an amputated thumb, toe transfers to the hand have become the standard for like-with-like reconstruction in thumb and finger deficits. In spite of the fact that it is now possible to treat multiple finger amputations, fingertip injuries, and traumatic or posttraumatic joint involvement, the reconstruction of the thumb continues to be the primary indication for toe transfer.[31]

Versatility of the Great Toe-to-Thumb Reconstruction

A wide variety of combinations gives the opportunity to plan a custom-made transfer that best adapts to specific situations. In cases where the proximal part of the thumb has been amputated, the question of whether to perform delayed or immediate reconstruction is one that is currently being discussed in the medical literature.[32–34]

Great Toe Transfer

The great toe transfer technique produces the best results when applied to thumb amputations performed through the proximal phalanx. Under these circumstances, the ROM in all three joints of the first ray is restored. Although the complete transfer of the great toe, including the metatarsophalangeal joint (MTPJ), has been advocated by some surgeons,[35] the morbidity of the donor site has made others abandon this technique.[36,37] Buncke and colleagues[35] reported the long-term results of 73 patients with a great toe transfer. The average motion of the metacarpophalangeal joint was 63% and the interphalangeal joint (IPJ) was 59% of the ROM on the opposite side. Grip strength was 77%, and pinch strength was 67% that of the uninjured side. In this series, most of the secondary procedures were performed to narrow the size of the great toe. Although the authors reported rare donor site problems, Barca and colleagues[38] found that the lack of the first MTPJ is responsible for lateral metatarsal and toe overload and destabilization in the final step phase.

Wrap-Around Technique

The wrap-around technique was described by Morrison and colleagues[39] with the aim of avoiding the bulkiness and donor site morbidity of the great toe transfer. This flap includes skin, nail, and pulp from the big toe, which wrap around an iliac crest bone graft. However, the non-vascularized bone graft has a frequent tendency to absorb.[40] Because of this, Morrison and colleagues[41] modified the technique by including a segment of the distal phalanx with the wrap-around flap. This was a technique that had already been presented by Foucher and colleagues[42] The wrap-around technique has been recommended for amputation distal to the thumb IPJ to preserve the nail pinch (**Fig. 2**).[36] Adani and colleagues[43] evaluated 10 patients with thumb amputation distal to or at the IPJ. Although they did not compare the results, those patients who retained the IPJ achieved a flexion–extension arc between 25° and 45°. The average amount of sensory recovery seen during the static two-point discrimination test was 10 mm.

Trimmed-Toe Technique

Wei and colleagues[44] published the description of the trimmed toe transfer procedure at the same time as Upton and Mutimer.[45] This procedure makes longitudinal osteotomy on the proximal and distal phalanges of the great toe to thin toe while preserving the IPJ. The indications are comparable to those of great toe transfer when the great toe demonstrates overall dimensions that are obviously larger than the thumb. To avoid the trimmed-joint itself becoming unstable, careful attention should be paid to the process of accurately reattaching the medial collateral ligament and the capsule of the interphalangeal joint of the great toe.[44]

Wei and colleagues[44] reported the results of 26 patients who underwent this technique. The IPJ motion averaged 18° (range 0° to 40°) in 11 patients who had no fusion of the IPJ. Although this technique has minimal interference with the function of the foot by leaving at least 1 cm of proximal phalanx, the appearance of the donor site is the main disadvantage. To overcome this problem, del Piñal and colleagues[46] published a technique to improve the foot's appearance after a trimmed-toe harvest by means of removing the second metatarsal and transposing the second toe on top of the hallux stump.

Twisted-Toe

In 1980, Foucher and colleagues[42] described the twisted-toe flap with the aim of building a custom-made new distal digit. In this technique, an onycho-cutaneous flap of the great toe, the tibial pulp of the second toe, and a piece of either the distal phalanx of the hallux or the second toe are harvested over the same vascular pedicle. Although Foucher and colleagues[42] described this technique for distal reconstructions in the thumb and fingers, Iglesias and colleagues[47] used this technique to reconstruct 12 patients with thumb amputation at the first phalanx or at the metacarpophalangeal level. Tsai and Aziz[48] modified the technique by combining the wrap-around flap from the great toe with a vascularized joint transfer, either the proximal interphalangeal joint (PIPJ) or the MTPJ of the second toe (**Fig. 3**). The advantage of this technique is that it is technically less demanding than the original twisted-toe technique because it avoids twisting the flap of the second toe, minimizing the risk of vascular complications. del Piñal,[49] in another modification, combined the trimmed-toe technique with the MTPJ of the second toe, a technique he defined as "switching-two-toe transfer."

Custom-Made Reconstructions

The great toe has been used to perform custom-made reconstructions in partial amputations not only in the thumb but also in the fingers. Foucher and colleagues[42] described the use of a partial transfer of the great toe to treat total and partial distal finger amputations. In total distal reconstruction, the nail matrix has to be harvested along with part of the pulp, a piece of bone, and the nail bed. On the contrary, in partial distal amputation, the flap does not include the nail matrix. Koshima and colleagues[50] presented the osteo-onycho-cutaneous flap of the hallux for reconstruction of the distal phalanx in the fingers in two cases. The main advantage of this technique is that it avoids amputation of the donor site, as in the case of using the second toe (**Fig. 4**). del Piñal and colleagues[51] reported the results of 25 patients, most of them manual workers, who suffered

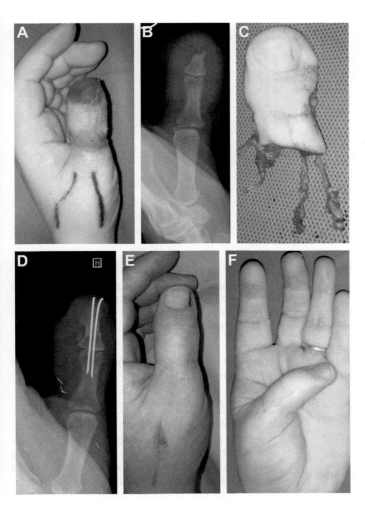

Fig. 2. (*A*) Amputation of the left thumb in a 34-year-old female patient. (*B*) The level of the amputation is distal to the IPJ. (*C*) Wrap-around flap harvested from the left foot. (*D*) Insetting of the flap with the distal phalanx fragment of the great toe. (*E*) Cosmetic result of the thumb. (*F*) Range of motion of the reconstructed thumb.

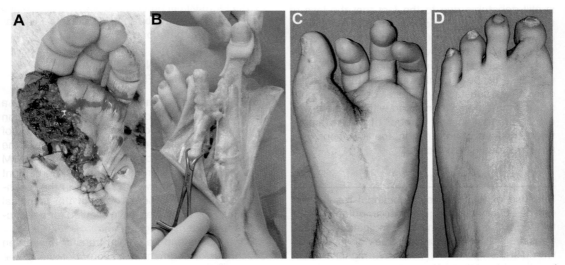

Fig. 3. (*A*) Severe crush injury of the left dominant hand in a 31-year-old male patient. (*B*) A twisted-toe procedure. (*C*) Result at 4 years of follow-up. Coverage of the proximal thumb and the first web space was with a lateral arm free flap. (*D*) The final result of the donor site.

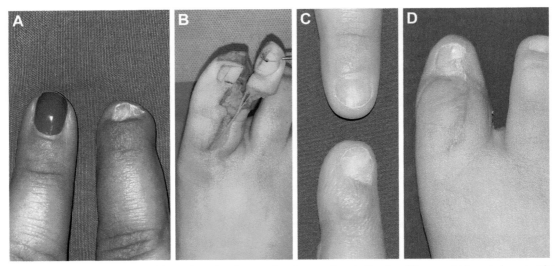

Fig. 4. (*A*) Distal amputation of the right index finger after 1 year of evolution in a 26-year-old female lawyer. The nail matrix was also injured, causing a dystrophic nail plate. (*B*) An osteo-onycho-cutaneous flap of the great toe was harvested for fingertip reconstruction. (*C*) Comparative result with the contralateral side (top). (*D*) At the donor site, it is possible to maintain the nail plate in all toes with this approach.

amputation of the thumb distal to the IPJ. At a minimum follow-up of 1 year, the Patient-Rated Wrist-Hand Evaluation (PRWHE) averaged 3.5, and the average American Orthopedic Foot and Ankle Society score was 94 of 100. All patients resumed their previous work without limitations 2 to 4.5 months after the operation.

SECOND AND THIRD TOE TRANSFERS FOR FINGER RECONSTRUCTION

Single-digit reconstruction with toe transplantation is still debatable due to the fact that the loss of functionality in the hand is relatively minor when only one finger is absent. However, in selected patients and in situations where optimal reconstruction is desired, a reconstruction of the finger using like-tissue transplanted from the foot typically offers satisfactory results. del Piñal[52] considers four factors when faced with a patient with digital amputation: the number of fingers amputated, the level of amputation, toe limitations, and a harmonious digital arcade.

Single Finger Amputation

Because of the excellent functional results that can be achieved, a single-finger amputation distal to the PIPJ is one of the best indications for toe transfer. This is particularly true for individuals with distal amputations who have higher manual functional or esthetic demands as a result of their occupation or hobbies (**Fig. 5**). On the other hand, a ray amputation is an effective treatment

option for a single-finger amputation that occurs proximal to this joint.[52,53]

Multiple Finger Amputations

When faced with even more devastating amputations that involve multiple fingers, the reconstructive plan becomes more complicated. The radial two digits play the most important role in global hand function, particularly during fine manipulation, and should be prioritized during reconstruction. However, a few patients have specific requirements for maximal hand span, and the ulnar digits may be of greater importance, particularly in metacarpal hand amputations.[54–56]

VASCULARIZED BONE, JOINT, AND OSTEOCHONDRAL FLAP

Vascularized joint transfer from the foot is a reasonable resource for finger joint reconstruction in young patients. Although the ROM of the PIPJ of the toe is less than its counterpart in the hand, the mobility obtained allows for a functional ROM (**Fig. 6**). However, there is widespread agreement that an extensor lag will be present in the reconstructed PIPJ. In general, none of the technical modifications described have allowed for a reduction in this extensor lag.[57,58]

Bone blocks and hemi-joint transfer have been described for segmental osseous defects of the fingers.[59] This approach allows for reconstruction of compound defects or septic nonunion in one stage (**Fig. 7**).

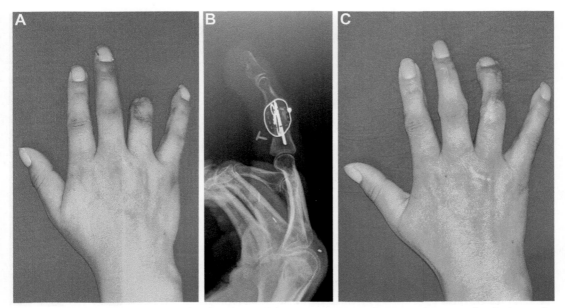

Fig. 5. (*A*) Single finger amputation distal to the IPJ. (*B*) Reconstruction with a second toe transfer. An intercalary bone graft (*red frame*) was used to avoid an unbalanced reconstruction. (*C*) The final result with an appropriate length.

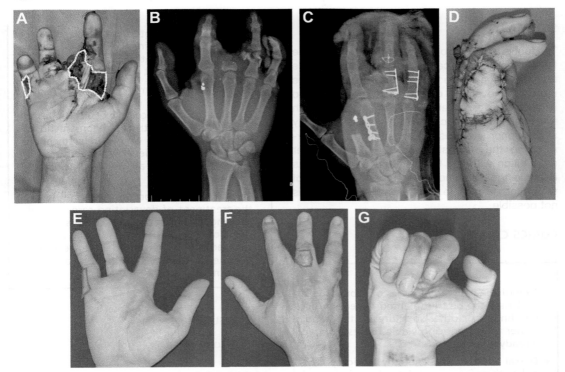

Fig. 6. (*A, B*) Severe injury with amputation of the long finger, skin defects of the volar base of the index and the ulnar side of the little finger (outlined in *white*), and PIPJ injury with osteochondral defect at the ring finger. (*C*) A third-ray amputation with second-ray transposition allowed closure of the volar skin defect of the index finger. A vascularized joint from the right second toe was used to reconstruct the osteochondral defect of the ring finger. (*D*) A skin only flow-through flap from the left second toe was used to cover the ulnar aspect of the little finger. (*E, F*) The final cosmetic result of the hand. The skin flap of the second toe (*E*) and the skin flap of the vascularized joint (*F*) are outlined in red. (*G*) Final result with an acceptable ROM of the fingers.

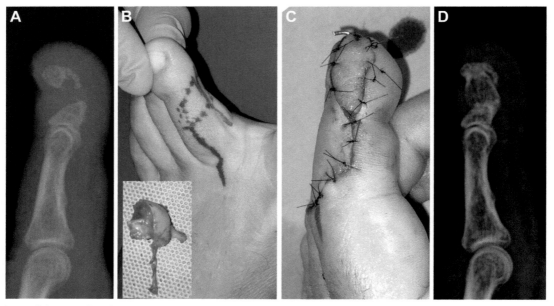

Fig. 7. (*A*) Intercalary bone defect of the distal phalanx of the index finger caused by a grinder machine in a manual worker. (*B*) An osteocutaneous bone flap was harvested from the middle phalanx of the second toe. (*C*) Insetting of the flap. (*D*) At 4 weeks postoperatively, bone union occurred, and he returned to work at 6 weeks.

SUMMARY

The foot is a unique source of reconstructive tissue for the hand. Surgical techniques allow for the reconstruction of like with like. These procedures require innovative, out-of-the-box thinking to achieve the desired end result of preserving both function and esthetics while reducing morbidity at the donor site. Despite some controversy surrounding the reconstruction of a single finger amputation with toe transfer, this treatment has become the best indication for amputations of the thumb or multiple fingers when replantation is not possible.

CLINICS CARE POINTS

- One of the main advantages of foot tissue is that they can be transplanted to reconstruct lost fingers or other structures in the hand, rather than sacrificing viable tissues from an already injured hand.
- Dorsal foot arterial anatomy is highly variable; therefore, complete knowledge of anatomic variants is essential when planning a reconstructive procedure.
- In relation to the pathway of the first plantar metatarsal artery, there are several classifications based on its relationship to the first dorsal interosseous muscle or its location at the depth of the first interosseous space. Nevertheless, the predominance of the dorsal variants over the plantar variants is constant among the different classifications.

- Techniques for thumb reconstruction using the great toe have evolved from complete transfer to more complex techniques, in which a more esthetic reconstruction is sought. The choice of the ideal technique will depend on the level of the defect at the level of the thumb as well as the surgeon's preference.

- Second and third toe transfers are useful in the treatment of devastating cases of multiple finger amputations. In these situations, the choice of which fingers should be reconstructed should be prioritized in relation to the specific activities the patient expects to perform afterward.

DISCLOSURES

Nothing to disclose.

REFERENCES

1. Cobbett JR. Free digital transfer. Report of a case of transfer of a great toe to replace an amputated thumb. J Bone Joint Surg Br 1969;51(4):677–9.
2. Buncke HJ Jr, Buncke CM, Schulz WP. Immediate Nicoladoni procedure in the Rhesus monkey, or

hallux-to-hand transplantation, utilising microminiature vascular anastomoses. Br J Plast Surg 1966; 19(4):332–7.

3. Fang F, Chung KC. An evolutionary perspective on the history of flap reconstruction in the upper extremity. Hand Clin 2014;30(2):109–22, v.

4. Taylor GI, Pan WR. Angiosomes of the leg: anatomic study and clinical implications. Plast Reconstr Surg 1998;102(3):599–616. discussion 617-618.

5. Lee JH, Dauber W. Anatomic study of the dorsalis pedis-first dorsal metatarsal artery. Ann Plast Surg 1997;38(1):50–5.

6. Hemamalini, Manjunatha HN. Variations in the origin, course and branching pattern of dorsalis pedis artery with clinical significance. Sci Rep 2021;11(1): 1448.

7. Villén GM, Julve GG. The Arterial System of the First Intermetatarsal Space and its Influence in Toe-To-Hand Transfer: A Report of 53 Long-Pedicle Transfers. J Hand Surg Am 2002;27(1):73–7.

8. Leung PC, Wong WL. The vessels of the first metatarsal web space. An operative and radiographic study. J Bone Joint Surg Am 1983;65(2):235–8.

9. Kim JW, Choi YJ, Lee HJ, et al. Anatomic Study of the Dorsalis Pedis Artery, First Metatarsal Artery, and Second Metatarsal Bone for Mandibular Reconstruction. J Oral Maxillofac Surg 2015;73(8): 1627–36.

10. Hou Z, Zou J, Wang Z, et al. Anatomical classification of the first dorsal metatarsal artery and its clinical application. Plast Reconstr Surg 2013;132(6): 1028e–39e.

11. Merle M, Dautel G, Loda G. Reconstruction du pouce. In: Merle M, Dautel G, editors. La main traumatique: chirurgie secondaire, le poignet traumatiquevol. 2. Paris: Elsevier Masson; 1995. p. 225–79.

12. May JW Jr, Chait LA, Cohen BE, et al. Free neurovascular flap from the first web of the foot in hand reconstruction. J Hand Surg Am 1977;2(5):387–93.

13. Spanio S, Wei FC, Coskunfirat OK, et al. Symmetry of Vascular Pedicle Anatomy in the First Web Space of the Foot Related to Toe Harvest: Clinical Observations in 85 Simultaneous Bilateral Second-Toe Transfer Patients. Plast Reconstr Surg 2005;115(5): 1325.

14. McCraw JB, Furlow LT Jr. The dorsalis pedis arterialized flap. A clinical study. Plast Reconstr Surg 1975; 55(2):177–85.

15. Samson MC, Morris SF, Tweed AE. Dorsalis pedis flap donor site: acceptable or not? Plast Reconstr Surg 1998;102(5):1549–54.

16. Zuker RM, Manktelow RT. The dorsalis pedis free flap: technique of elevation, foot closure, and flap application. Plast Reconstr Surg 1986;77(1):93–104.

17. Ono S, Sebastin SJ, Ohi H, et al. Microsurgical Flaps in Repair and Reconstruction of the Hand. Hand Clin 2017;33(3):425–41.

18. Chung KC, Tong L. Use of three free flaps based on a single vascular pedicle for complex hand reconstruction in an electrical burn injury: a case report. J Hand Surg Am 2001;26(5):956–61.

19. Eo S, Kim Y, Kim JYS, et al. The versatility of the dorsalis pedis compound free flap in hand reconstruction. Ann Plast Surg 2008;61(2):157–63.

20. Hallock GG. Further clarification of the nomenclature for compound flaps. Plast Reconstr Surg 2006; 117(7):151e–60e.

21. Xie G, Hu Z, Miao C, et al. The free triple chimeric dorsalis pedis flaps for repair of multifinger soft tissue defects: a report of two cases. Microsurgery 2013;33(8):660–6.

22. Desai SS, Chuang DC, Levin LS. Microsurgical reconstruction of the extensor system. Hand Clin 1995;11(3):471–82.

23. Adani R, Marcoccio I, Tarallo L. Flap coverage of dorsum of hand associated with extensor tendons injuries: A completely vascularized single-stage reconstruction. Microsurgery 2003;23(1):32–9.

24. Cho BC, Lee JH, Weinzweig N, et al. Use of the free innervated dorsalis pedis tendocutaneous flap in composite hand reconstruction. Ann Plast Surg 1998;40(3):268–76.

25. Coulet B, Boretto JG, Lazerges C, et al. « Mains de portière » : classification lésionnelle et stratégie thérapeutique. Chir Main 2011;30(4):246–54.

26. del Piñal F, Herrero F. Extensor digitorum brevis free flap: anatomic study and further clinical applications. Plast Reconstr Surg 2000;105(4):1347–56.

27. Hallock GG. The conjoint extensor digitorum brevis muscle and dorsalis pedis osteocutaneous island flap. Ann Plast Surg 1990;24(4):371–7.

28. Zhu SX, Zhang BX, Yao JX, et al. Free Musculocutaneous Flap Transfer of Extensor Digitorum Brevis Muscle by Microvascular Anastomosis for Restoration of Function of Thenar and Adductor Pollicis Muscles. Ann Plast Surg 1985;15(6):481.

29. Mitz V. Second toe to thumb transfer with extensor digitorum brevis opponensplasty. Ann Plast Surg 1986;17(3):259–62.

30. Tamai S, Fukui A, Shimizu T, et al. Thumb reconstruction with an iliac bone graft and a dorsalis pedis flap transplant including the extensor digitorum brevis muscle for restoring opposition: a case report. Microsurgery 1983;4(2):81–6.

31. Waljee JF, Chung KC. Toe-to-hand transfer: evolving indications and relevant outcomes. J Hand Surg Am 2013;38(7):1431–4.

32. Del Piñal F. Reply: Extreme Thumb Losses: Reconstructive Strategies. Plast Reconstr Surg 2020; 145(5):1007e–8e.

33. Lin CH, Mardini S, Lin YT, et al. Osteoplastic thumb ray restoration with or without secondary toe transfer for reconstruction of opposable basic hand function. Plast Reconstr Surg 2008;121(4):1288–97.

34. Kempny T, Paroulek J, Marik V, et al. Further developments in the twisted-toe technique for isolated thumb reconstruction: our method of choice. Plast Reconstr Surg 2013;131(6):871e–9e.

35. Buncke GM, Buncke HJ, Lee CK. Great toe-to-thumb microvascular transplantation after traumatic amputation. Hand Clin 2007;23(1):105–15.

36. Wei FC, Chen HC, Chuang CC, et al. Microsurgical thumb reconstruction with toe transfer: selection of various techniques. Plast Reconstr Surg 1994; 93(2):345–51. discussion 352-357.

37. Foucher G, Binhammer P. Plea to save the great toe in total thumb reconstruction. Microsurgery 1995; 16(6):373–6.

38. Barca F, Santi A, Tartoni PL, et al. Gait analysis of the donor foot in microsurgical reconstruction of the thumb. Foot Ankle Int 1995;16(4):201–6.

39. Morrison WA, O'Brien BM, MacLeod AM. Thumb reconstruction with a free neurovascular wrap-around flap from the big toe. J Hand Surg Am 1980;5(6):575–83.

40. Leung PC, Ma FY. Digital reconstruction using the toe flap– report of 10 cases. J Hand Surg Am 1982;7(4):366–70.

41. Morrison WA, O'Brien BM, MacLeod AM. Experience with thumb reconstruction. J Hand Surg Br 1984;9(3):223–33.

42. Foucher G, Merle M, Maneaud M, et al. Microsurgical free partial toe transfer in hand reconstruction: a report of 12 cases. Plast Reconstr Surg 1980; 65(5):616–27.

43. Adani R, Cardon LJ, Castagnetti C, et al. Distal thumb reconstruction using a mini wrap-around flap from the great toe. J Hand Surg Br 1999;24(4): 437–42.

44. Wei FC, Chen HC, Chuang CC, et al. Reconstruction of the thumb with a trimmed-toe transfer technique. Plast Reconstr Surg 1988;82(3):506–15.

45. Upton J, Mutimer K. A modification of the great-toe transfer for thumb reconstruction. Plast Reconstr Surg 1988;82(3):535–8.

46. del Piñal F, García-Bernal FJ, Regalado J, et al. A technique to improve foot appearance after trimmed toe or hallux harvesting. J Hand Surg Am 2007;32(3):409–13.

47. Iglesias M, Butron P, Serrano A. Thumb reconstruction with extended twisted toe flap. J Hand Surg Am 1995;20(5):731–6.

48. Tsai TM, Aziz W. Toe-to-thumb transfer: a new technique. Plast Reconstr Surg 1991;88(1):149–53.

49. Del Piñal F. Extreme Thumb Losses: Reconstructive Strategies. Plast Reconstr Surg 2019;144(3):665–77.

50. Koshima I, Ohno A, Yamasaki M. Free Vascularized Osteo-Onychocutaneous Flap for Reconstruction of the Distal Phalanx of the Fingers. J Reconstr Microsurg 1989;5(04):337–42.

51. Del Piñal F, Moraleda E, de Piero GH, et al. Onycho-osteo-cutaneous defects of the thumb reconstructed by partial hallux transfer. J Hand Surg Am 2014; 39(1):29–36.

52. del Piñal F. The indications for toe transfer after "minor" finger injuries. J Hand Surg Br 2004;29(2):120–9.

53. del Piñal F, Herrero F, García-Bernal FJ, et al. Minimizing impairment in laborers with finger losses distal to the proximal interphalangeal joint by second toe transfer. Plast Reconstr Surg 2003;112(4): 1000–11.

54. Wei FC, Epstein MD, Chen HC, et al. Microsurgical reconstruction of distal digits following mutilating hand injuries: results in 121 patients. Br J Plast Surg 1993;46(3):181–6.

55. Wallace CG, Wei FC. Posttraumatic finger reconstruction with microsurgical transplantation of toes. Hand Clin 2007;23(1):117–28.

56. Wei FC, el-Gammal TA, Lin CH, et al. Metacarpal hand: classification and guidelines for microsurgical reconstruction with toe transfers. Plast Reconstr Surg 1997;99(1):122–8.

57. Tsubokawa N, Yoshizu T, Maki Y. Long-term results of free vascularized second toe joint transfers to finger proximal interphalangeal joints. J Hand Surg Am 2003;28(3):443–7.

58. Dautel G. Vascularized toe joint transfers to the hand for PIP or MCP reconstruction. Hand Surg Rehabil 2018;37(6):329–36.

59. del Piñal F, García-Bernal FJ, Delgado J, et al. Vascularized bone blocks from the toe phalanx to solve complex intercalated defects in the fingers. J Hand Surg Am 2006;31(7):1075–82.

Functional Free Muscle Transfer for Reconstruction of Traumatic Adult Brachial Plexus Injuries

Raquel Bernardelli Iamaguchi, MD, MSc, PhD*,
Marcelo Rosa de Rezende, MD, PhD

KEYWORDS

- Free muscle transfer • Brachial plexus • Paralysis • Gracilis transfer • Elbow flexion reconstruction
- Functional outcome

KEY POINTS

- Functional free muscle transfer (FFMT) for adult brachial plexus reconstruction is one of the most challenging and demanding techniques in reconstructive microsurgery.
- FFMT for traumatic brachial plexus injuries (BPI) requires technical standardization to facilitate faster surgery and reduce factors influencing the success of functional outcomes.
- Precise microsurgical technique must be complemented by mechanical stability to obtain greater FFMT strength.
- The choice of donor nerve is the key for a successful FFMT; be sure of function and avoid nerve grafts.
- A long rehabilitation process is expected, even for a motivated patient.

 Video content accompanies this article at http://www.hand.theclinics.com.

INTRODUCTION

Adult brachial plexus injuries (BPI) are devastating injuries that affect more commonly young adults, resulting in permanent sequelae, which affect work and daily life activities. The severe physical and psychological disability, as well as the costs to the health system throughout the life of a young adult justifies using all the surgical options available, including one of the most demanding techniques in microsurgery, the free functional muscle transfer (FFMT). Elbow flexion is a priority in upper extremity functional recovery in BPI[1] and FFMT for elbow flexion is a workhorse in selected BPI cases.

Treatment options for adult BPI include nerve grafts if nerve roots are available, vascularized nerve grafts and nerve transfers. In severe cases of total BPI, no functional recovery after brachial plexus surgery and late presentation, when neurologic reconstruction is no longer possible, the FFMT is the best option. We can extrapolate the concept of the reconstructive elevator, described by Gottlieb and colleagues[2] for wound-closure, to achieve better functional results in adult BPI with FFMT for elbow flexion or double FFMT for total BPI, as the first line of treatment.[3] The FFMT can be indicated as a definitive and immediate upper limb reconstruction surgery in selected cases, when nerve roots are not adequate or unavailable

Hand Surgery and Reconstructive Microsurgery Group of the Institute of Orthopedics and Traumatology, Clinics Hospital of University of Sao Paulo, São Paulo, Brazil
* Corresponding author. Rua Dr. Ovídio Pires de Campos, 333, Sao Paulo, São Paulo 05403-010, Brazil.
E-mail address: rbiamaguchi@gmail.com

Hand Clin 40 (2024) 259–267
https://doi.org/10.1016/j.hcl.2023.08.011
0749-0712/24/© 2023 Elsevier Inc. All rights reserved.

for reconstruction or late cases 12 months or more from injury.[4]

The use of FFMT in BPI must be encouraged to allow consistent functional results for reanimation of the upper extremity, especially for elbow flexion.[5] This review will discuss data available for FFMT in adult traumatic BPI, technical recommendations and future directions to achieve better functional results for the reanimation of a paralytic upper limb.

CLINICAL ASSESSMENT

Stevanovic and Sharpe[6] describe the requirements for patient selection for FFMT, including patient motivation and collaboration for postoperative rehabilitation. They recommend that FFMT should not be performed in patients with comorbidities such as diabetes, peripheral vascular disease, autoimmune disease, and smoking. Although, we consider comorbidities as risk factors for complications and not a contraindication for FFMT.

There is no recommended age limit to perform FFMT, although authors[6] have recommended 45 years or less for FFMT. Doi and colleagues[7] reported FFMT for extremity reconstruction and described that reinnervation results for BPI were not influenced by age. Suroto and colleagues[8] studied FFMT for elbow flexion and did not observe a correlation between age and BMI with functional outcomes or range of motion (ROM), although the average age was 27.71 ± 10.63. Similar results are described by Steendam and colleagues[9] with an average age of 23 years, demonstrating that the chronologic age is not a contraindication for microsurgery. Epidemiologically, patients with adult BPI are young with a mean age of 30 years or less. Hence, age is not a concern during patient selection for FFMT and even age more than 45 years should not be a contraindication for FFMT in motivated patients and with good rehabilitation support.

Brophy and Wolfe[1] described an incidence of 75% of patients with supraclavicular injuries. In these patients, 50% had total paralysis. The incidence of infraclavicular injuries was 25%; within this group, 45% of patients had total paralysis. Alnot described a similar distribution,[10] with 75% having supraclavicular lesions and 75% to 80% with total BPI (C5-T1). Total paralysis and partial upper BPI are responsible for more than 90% of adult BPI. In both injuries, there is functional loss of elbow flexion that is the priority for reconstruction in BPI surgeries.

The physical examination is the key to decision-making for reconstruction. Narakas and colleagues[11] observed that 10% of patients had combined supraclavicular and infraclavicular lesions. Qiu SS[12] and colleagues identified clinical predictors for infraclavicular BPI: presence of a healthy clavicular head of pectoralis major or biceps, scapular fracture, and infraclavicular tinel sign. Limthongthang and colleagues[13] in a review article described the advantages of further subdividing preganglionic and postganglionic injury as a prognostic value.

IMAGING

MRI for traumatic adult BPI is the imaging technique of choice (**Fig. 1**), with the advantage of being less invasive than computed tomography myelography.[14] MRI is easily able to identify a preganglionic lesion with a pseudomeningocele in MRI T2-weighted images with an attenuated or disrupted nerve root or spinal cord signal intensity changes,[15] or spinal cord dislocation inside the cervical canal after root avulsion. Pseudomeningocele is not pathognomonic of a preganglionic lesion because it may happen without nerve avulsion.[16] However, in these cases, the nerve roots even if not completely avulsed are usually not adequate for nerve reconstruction with graft.

New developments in MRI for traumatic BPI include high-definition imaging for preganglionic and postganglionic injuries and combination of MRI with ultrasound.[17]

WHAT CLINICAL AND IMAGING FACTORS ARE IMPORTANT FOR FUNCTIONAL FREE MUSCLE TRANSFER FOR BRACHIAL PLEXUS INJURY RECONSTRUCTION?

One common concern is whether the recovered intraplexal nerve in BPI is strong enough to be a nerve source for FFMT, and this decision needs to be supported by physical examination and complementary examinations such as eletrodiagnostic studies.[18] For patients with a recovered intraplexal nerve with Medical Research Council (MRC) scale of muscle strength M4-or less, we prefer to use a noninjured donor nerve from extraplexal sources.

The other common indication for FFMT is a patient with failure of previous BPI surgery. Preoperative planning should include further investigation about recipient vessels and additional angiography should provide information on the best recipient artery and the adequate level to perform the microanastomosis outside the lesion and area of previous surgery.[19]

Time to Surgery

Traditionally, surgery in traumatic BPI was performed after 6 months in the absence of recovery

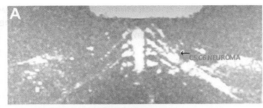
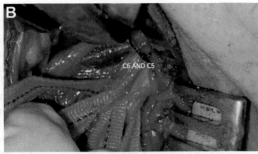
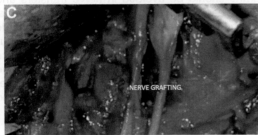

Fig. 1. (*A*) MRI with postganglionic injury of C5 and C6 roots; (*B*) intraoperative exploration showing C5 and C6 roots with intact proximal stump and distal neuroma similar to MRI image; and (*C*) reconstruction with sural nerve grafts.

of elbow flexion.[20] Although, in total traumatic BPI with limited extraplexal donor nerves and severe avulsion injury, the double FFMT described by Doi and colleagues[7] can be performed in the acute phase, less than 3 to 6 months for elbow flexion and finger extension (first FFMT), followed by FFMT for finger flexion (second FFMT). Barrie and colleagues[21] described double FFMT combined with triceps neurotization.

Although the most common indication for FFMT to restore elbow flexion is total BPI, FFMT often is indicated after a failed nerve reconstruction for traumatic adult BPI. In cases after more than 6 months from injury, FFMT would be preferable for elbow flexion instead of intercostal nerve (ICN) neurotization for elbow flexion, which can have variable results.[22]

Absence of elbow flexion impairs outcomes of reconstruction. Estrella and colleagues[23] observed in a cross-sectional study that quality of life through the evaluation of disabilities of arm, shoulder and Hand (DASH) score was positively affected by

higher range of motion following recovery of elbow flexion.

Secondary or early reconstruction with functional free muscle transfer

Factors affecting decision for FFMT include the following: (1) time elapsed between the injury and initial treatment and (2) absence of viable reconstructable nerve roots. The decision on when to perform the FFMT—after more than 12 months of injury or at the first stage of adult BPI reconstruction—is still a controversial topic in the published literature. Griepp and colleagues[24] in a systematic review found higher MRC strength scores for FFMT compared with non–free flap procedures including vascularized ulnar nerve graft, nerve transfers (Oberlin, intercostal to musculocutaneous), Steindler flexorplasty, and pedicled flaps. Chuang and colleagues[25] reported similar results of FFMT for restoration of elbow flexion when compared with Latissimus dorsi transfer. Although, depending on injury type and location, the Latissimus dorsi is usually either not available for transfer in adult BPI or not strong enough for nonvascularized transfer.

Giuffre and colleagues[26] described in a review article that each patient has a unique pattern of nerve injury; therefore, it is difficult to propose an algorithm for adult BPI.

In a systematic review, Hoang and colleagues[4] compared FFMT and nerve reconstruction for elbow flexion in patients with late presentation within 12 to 18 months of traumatic BPI. Results were superior with FFMT for elbow flexion, when compared with nerve grafting or nerve transfers.

Hence, when considering an algorithm for early use of FFMT (**Fig. 2**), selected cases may be considered less than 3 to 6 months from injury, which may result in better functional results in adult BPI.

Recipient Vessels

In FFMT for elbow flexion, the most common recipient vessels are the thoracoacromial vessels. Although, in previously failed reconstruction of adult BPI, there may be too much scarring at the recipient site and alternative recipient artery options are the thoracodorsal artery, branches of axillary artery or branches of brachial artery. Another option is to perform a reverse FFMT for elbow flexion with anastomosis to the radial artery and venae comitantes.[27] The caliber of the vessels and their compatibility with the vessels of the flap are also aspects to be considered. When the axillary branch anterior circumflex artery and veins are chosen as recipients, the pedicle is too short, which makes the anastomosis difficult. In addition,

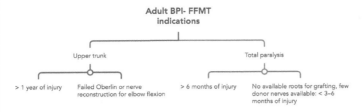

Fig. 2. Indications of FFMT for elbow flexion in adult BPI according to time elapsed from injury.

it is too distant from one of the most common donor nerves, the spinal accessory nerve (SAN). Therefore, a different approach including proximal attachment must be planned preoperatively.

The thoracodorsal pedicle, however, can be considered as a rescue option in exceptional cases, in which there are no other options— because its dissection and transposition to an area close to the pedicle of the flap is a more laborious procedure.

Our preference has been for the thoracoacromial pedicle, considering its favorable location for performing the anastomoses, a pedicle of adequate length and caliber, and compatibility with the vascular pedicle of the gracilis muscle flap. It is important that next to this pedicle, we have the cephalic vein, which despite its larger dimensions, can be used in cases, in which there is a larger vein from the gracilis pedicle.

A vascular imaging study of the affected limb is only justified if a vascular injury is suspected in patients with high-energy trauma with multiple injuries, usually associated with clavicle, scapular, or rib fractures.

The number of veins may influence results. Therefore, it is recommendable to perform 2 veins for drainage instead of only one vein.[28] We prefer to use one recipient vein from the deep system (*venae comitantes* of the chosen recipient artery) and, whenever possible, another vein from the superficial system, most commonly, the cephalic vein.

Donor Nerve

There are many donor nerve options for neurotization targeting elbow flexion: phrenic,[10] thoracodorsal, contralateral medial pectoral, ICN, SAN, contralateral C7, median, and ulnar nerves. Some authors describe better functional results with intraplexal nerves that are closer to the target FFMT.[29]

In partial brachial plexus injuries, SAN, ulnar, and median nerves may be used. In an article published by our group,[30] we observed better results with SAN but these were not statistically superior to results using an ulnar nerve fascicle as the donor nerve. It is possible that the intraplexal

donor nerve may be initially affected by the traumatic lesion and may not be fully recovered and hence might not be good options even in partial BPI. In partial BPI, Coulet and colleagues[31] described good results in all cases of FFMT for elbow flexion, reinnervated with third, fourth, and fifth ICNs.

In the literature, there is a consensus that nerve grafts should be avoided in nerve transfers and FFMT because it can result in a worse functional recovery. Therefore, every effort should be made to obtain the greatest possible length of the obturator nerve as well as the donor nerve. The choice is affected by previous surgeries as well as the type of paralysis (total or partial), and multicenter studies should provide statistical relevance and help microsurgeons in this decision.

SURGICAL TECHNIQUES/APPROACH
Proximal Insertion

The proximal muscle insertion of the FFMT depends on the site of microvascular anastomosis and donor nerves. When the recipient vessels are the thoracoacromial vessels, the gracilis can be proximally fixated through bone anchors or transosseous fixation in the distal third of clavicle or the acromion. When the donor nerve is the intercostals and when the recipient vessels are the thoracodorsal artery and vein, the FFMT can be fixated at the ribs or in the middle third of the clavicle. When the recipient vessels are a branch of the axillary or brachial artery and venae comitantes, the FFMT can be alternatively fixated at the coracoid process, if the muscle is overtensioned when attempting to reach the clavicle.

After the proximal fixation, the FFMT is passed distally through a subcutaneous tunnel or an open skin incision. An extensile incision may be necessary due to previous scarring in the arm or even individual physical characteristics, and skin grafting over the gracilis muscle may be necessary in these cases.

Distal Insertion

There is no conclusion in the literature about the ideal distal tendon attachment and options include

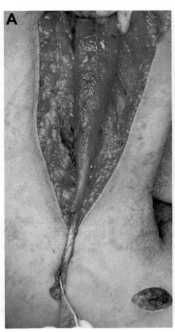
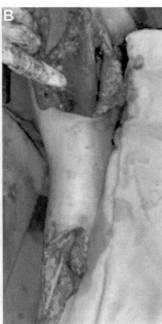

Fig. 3. (*A*) Marking the gracilis flap and (*B*) passing the gracilis through a tunnel at the arm, difficult visualization of the marked stitches.

the following[9]: distal biceps tendon, extensor carpi radialis brevis, extensor digitorum communis with extensor pollicis longus, and flexor digitorum profundus and flexor pollicis longus (FDP/FPL). Bertelli and colleagues[27] described a reverse gracilis FFMT with distal tendon insertion in acromion and muscle belly of gracilis sutured to the distal biceps. Traditionally, the distal insertion in our service is a Pulvertaft suture of gracilis tendon to distal biceps tendon and tension adjustment is a very important step. As described in the literature,[32] the gracilis flap can be marked with sutures at 1 cm intervals before it is detached from the thigh to help the surgeon to recover the adequate tension. However, this step may not be useful when a subcutaneous tunnel between proximal and anterior elbow incisions is made to pass the gracilis muscle through the arm (**Fig. 3**). Video 1 shows tensioning of the FFMT.

Does the principle of a single muscle or tendon to provide a single function really apply to traumatic BPI? Referencing the first description of double FFMT for BPI by Doi and colleagues,[33] when the first-stage gracilis provides double functions including elbow flexion and fingers extension with wrist extensors as a pulley, it was proved that one muscle can provide more than one function. However, our experience shows that the second function has limited strength and usually reaches only M2 or M3, or functions through tenodesis. Alternatively, the second gracilis tendon attachment may be performed later

with tendon graft if FFMT achieves a good functional result.

Considering biomechanics, the ideal distal insertion of the FFMT should provide a high torque (muscular strength MRC at least 3–4), minimum track distortion (no bowstringing of the FFMT), without unnecessary change in direction (FFMT traction through the distal tendon should be linear vs multiple distal insertions). Maldonado and colleagues[34] studied FFMT for elbow flexion and observed significantly better functional results, including M3 or M4 elbow flexion and range of motion when the gracilis was attached more distally to FDP/FPL tendons compared with a biceps tendon attachment.

We would like to describe a technique of distal bone attachment of gracilis tendon to the radial tuberosity with a biotenodesis screw (donated by Arthrex), similar to the technique described by Terzis and Kostopoulos.[35] In our opinion, inserting the gracilis tendon directly into the bone reduces the loss of indirect traction when inserting into the biceps tendon. Moreover, the biceps tendon can be used as a pulley for the gracilis, transforming the gracilis FFMT into a new independent elbow flexor, which could provide a greater elbow flexion torque (**Fig. 4**).

Two cases were performed by the authors with traumatic adult BPI. Indications for FFMT were as follows: (1) late reconstruction of adult BPI, more than 2 years from injury and (2) failed reconstruction of BPI referred from another Hospital (**Fig. 5**).

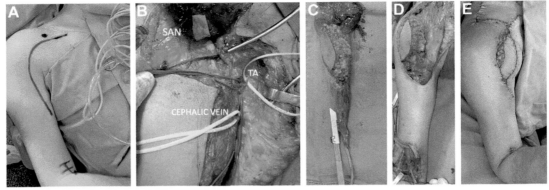

Fig. 4. A 30-year-old man after a motorcycle accident presented with an upper arm brachial plexus injury. (*A*) preoperative planning and marking of incisions, (*B*) donor nerve and recipient vessels preparation, (*C*) gracilis muscle flap, (*D*) anastomosis and neurotization with proximal gracilis muscle attached to clavicle with bone anchors and sutures, and (*E*) final distal suture of gracilis tendon with pulley through distal biceps and final insertion in radial tuberosity with transosseous suture.

Patients underwent gracilis FFMT for elbow flexion. Donor nerve for gracilis reinnervation was spinal accessory in both cases. The gracilis was distally attached without tendon graft after using the distal biceps tendon as a pulley and with direct bone attachment immediately distal to the radial tuberosity, using a similar technique to distal biceps tendon ruptures. This creates with the gracilis FFMT, a new elbow flexor muscle with traction in a straight line.

Surgical Recommendation

FFMT is a procedure that demands synchronization of 2 surgical teams, reducing the flap ischemia time and the total operative time.

One team prepares both the recipient area, identifying adequate recipient vessels and donor nerves, and the distal insertion site. Simultaneously, the other team prepares the gracilis muscle and pedicle with a maximal length. However, in cases with previous BPI surgery, we prefer to divide the surgery into 2 steps: first exploring for recipient vessels and donor nerves, followed by preparation of the gracilis muscle flap.

Before clamping the gracilis vessels, adequate length of vascular pedicle and donor nerve should be confirmed and necessary adjustments with the FFMT insertion site should be performed. This routine aims to minimize the ischemia time of the gracilis muscle, reducing damage to the muscle fibers and potentially improving functional outcomes of FFMT for elbow flexion.[28]

The functional rehabilitation process of the FFMT must be performed by a specialized therapist. After 21 days, light passive exercises are allowed with mobilization of the shoulder and elbow, with special attention to avoid extension of the elbow beyond 90°. After 6 weeks, the

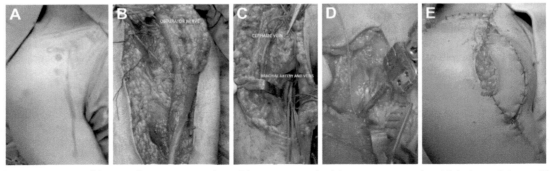

Fig. 5. A 36-year-old man after a motorcycle accident presented with an upper arm brachial plexus injury with failed Oberlin and nerve graft reconstruction referred for FFMT surgery for elbow flexion. (*A*) preoperative planning and marking of incisions, (*B*) gracilis muscle flap, (*C*) brachial artery/veins and cephalic vein, (*D*) distal insertion of gracilis tendon in radial tuberosity with biotenodesis screw, pulley through distal biceps tendon, and (*E*) after flap inset.

therapy progresses to full arc of movement and initial training focused on cortical plasticity of the transferred nerve.

The functional success of the transfers largely depends on the patient's motivation and cooperation in rehabilitation. The beginning of the reinnervation of the gracilis muscle starts around 3 months and can continue up to 2 years, requiring continuing rehabilitation and training (Video 2). With early signals of muscle contraction, the patient is encouraged to perform strengthening without gravity, beginning exercises in the horizontal plane until the patient is able to perform exercises against gravity, when the patient is encouraged to stop using the sling (Video 3).

Clinical Outcomes

The result of the FFMT surgery must be seen from the perspective of the patient's preoperative absence of function, especially in patients with total adult BPI with late presentation. This presents a functional challenge and even with suboptimal results with M3 strength of elbow flexion, the FFMT function represents an important gain for daily life activities and may allow the patient to return to work.

In our experience, SAN as the donor nerve is the best option, based on compatibility of nerve axon counts and synergistic contraction of elbow flexion with the trapezius muscle. With ICN as the donor nerve, a longer rehabilitation process is expected. Patients may initially have difficulty dissociating deep inspiration from elbow flexion but results may be seen up to 2 years after surgery (Video 4).

Orthopedic surgeries such as wrist arthrodesis and eventually shoulder arthrodesis or transfer of the upper trapezius for shoulder abduction should be considered to aid limb stability and help the FFMT for elbow flexion to achieve its full contractile capacity. Doi and colleagues[36] described that upper limb reconstructed with FFMT requires stability of the shoulder. Preserved shoulder mobility has better functional results compared with shoulder arthrodesis and should be considered with suprascapular nerve reconstruction when the serratus anterior (reconstructed or not injured) is functioning.

In partial upper adult BPI, with insufficient FFMT recovery (elbow flexion grades M3 or M2), Steindler flexorplasty can be a complementary surgery, with potential gain of 2° on the MRC scale.

At the end of these procedures, we will have a stable limb, with the possibility of improving body expression and allowing activities of daily living, reducing health-care costs for these debilitating injuries.

SUMMARY

There is a possibility that advances in nerve transfers and especially distal nerve transfers may reduce the indications of FFMT for elbow flexion and hand reanimation. However, in failed cases of nerve transfers or late presentation of adult BPI, FFMT for upper limb reconstruction is a reliable choice.

FFMT for adult BPI is time consuming for the patient and medical team; therefore, precise indications for this surgery must occur with good patient motivation. Better results with FFMT for adult BPI are expected with research advances for ideal donor nerves, robotic-assisted microsurgery,[37] and mechanical engineering assisting in determining the ideal surgical technique to achieve the best functional result.

CLINICS CARE POINTS

- FFMT for adult brachial plexus reconstruction is one of the most challenging and demanding techniques in reconstructive microsurgery.
- FFMT for traumatic BPI requires critical technical points to facilitate faster surgery and reduce factors influencing the success of functional outcomes.
- The donor muscle needs to be the workhorse muscle flap for each surgeon.
- The choice of donor nerve is the most important step; be sure of function and avoid nerve grafts.

DISCLOSURE

The authors have nothing to disclose.

SUPPLEMENTARY DATA

Supplementary data related to this article can be found online at https://doi.org/10.1016/j.hcl.2023.08.011.

REFERENCES

1. Brophy RH, Wolfe SW. Planning brachial plexus surgery: treatment options and priorities. Hand Clin 2005;21(1):47–54.
2. Gottlieb LJ, Krieger LM. From the reconstructive ladder to the reconstructive elevator. Plast Reconstr Surg 1994;93(7):1503–4.
3. Maldonado AA, Poppler L, Loosbrock Rn MF, et al. Restoration of Grasp after Single-Stage Free

Functioning Gracilis Muscle Transfer in Traumatic Adult Pan-Brachial Plexus Injury. Plast Reconstr Surg 2023;151(1):133–42.

4. Hoang D, Chen VW, Seruya M. Recovery of Elbow Flexion after Nerve Reconstruction versus Free Functional Muscle Transfer for Late, Traumatic Brachial Plexus Palsy: A Systematic Review. Plast Reconstr Surg 2018;141(4):949–59.

5. Kay S, Pinder R, Wiper J, et al. Microvascular free functioning gracilis transfer with nerve transfer to establish elbow flexion. J Plast Reconstr Aesthet Surg 2010;63(7):1142–9.

6. Stevanovic M, Sharpe F. Functional free muscle transfer for upper extremity reconstruction. Plast Reconstr Surg 2014;134(2):257e–74e.

7. Doi K, Sakai K, Ihara K, et al. Reinnervated free muscle transplantation for extremity reconstruction. Plast Reconstr Surg 1993;91(5):872–83.

8. Suroto H, Wardhani IL, Haryadi RD, et al. The Relationship Between Patient Factors and Clinical Outcomes of Free Functional Muscle Transfer in Patients with Complete Traumatic Brachial Plexus Injury. Orthop Res Rev 2022;14:225–33.

9. Steendam TC, Nelissen RGHH, Malessy MJA, et al. What is the Elbow Flexion Strength After Free Functional Gracilis Muscle Transfer for Adult Traumatic Complete Brachial Plexus Injuries? Clin Orthop Relat Res 2022;480(12):2392–405.

10. Alnot JY. Traumatic brachial plexus lesions in the adult. Indications and results. Hand Clin 1995;11(4):623–31.

11. Narakas AO. The treatment of brachial plexus injuries. Int Orthop 1985;9(1):29–36.

12. Qiu SS, Chang TN, Lu JC, et al. Reliability of Various Predictors for Preoperative Diagnosis of Infraclavicular Brachial Plexus Lesions with Shoulder and/or Elbow Paresis. J Reconstr Microsurg 2020;36(6):445–9.

13. Limthongthang R, Bachoura A, Songcharoen P, et al. Adult brachial plexus injury: evaluation and management. Orthop Clin North Am 2013;44(4):591–603.

14. Caranci F, Briganti F, La Porta M, et al. Magnetic resonance imaging in brachial plexus injury. Musculoskelet Surg 2013;97(Suppl 2):S181–90.

15. Van Es HW, Bollen TL, van Heesewijk HP. MRI of the brachial plexus: a pictorial review. Eur J Radiol 2010;74(2):391–402.

16. Yoshikawa T, Hayashi N, Yamamoto S, et al. Brachial plexus injury: clinical manifestations, conventional imaging findings, and the latest imaging techniques. Radiographics 2006;26(Suppl 1):S133–43.

17. Koneru S, Nguyen VT, Hacquebord JH, et al. Brachial Plexus Nerve Injuries and Disorders: MR Imaging-Ultrasound Correlation. Magn Reson Imaging Clin N Am 2023 May;31(2):255–67.

18. Terzis JK, Kostopoulos VK. The surgical treatment of brachial plexus injuries in adults. Plast Reconstr Surg 2007;119(4):73e–92e.

19. Macedo LS, Rusig RP, Silva GB, et al. Computed tomography angiography and microsurgical flaps for traumatic wounds: What is the added value? Clin Hemorheol Microcirc 2021;78(3):237–45.

20. Noland SS, Bishop AT, Spinner RJ, et al. Adult Traumatic Brachial Plexus Injuries. J Am Acad Orthop Surg 2019;27(19):705–16.

21. Barrie KA, Steinmann SP, Shin AY, et al. Gracilis free muscle transfer for restoration of function after complete brachial plexus avulsion. Neurosurg Focus 2004;16(5):E8.

22. Terzis JK, Vekris MD, Soucacos PN. Outcomes of brachial plexus reconstruction in 204 patients with devastating paralysis. Plast Reconstr Surg 1999;104(5):1221–40.

23. Estrella EP, Castillo-Carandang NT, Cordero CP, et al. Quality of life of patients with traumatic brachial plexus injuries. Injury 2021;52(4):855–61.

24. Griepp DW, Shah NV, Scollan JP, et al. Outcomes of gracilis free-flap muscle transfers and non-free-flap procedures for restoration of elbow flexion: A systematic review. J Plast Reconstr Aesthet Surg 2022;75(8):2625–36.

25. Chuang DC, Epstein MD, Yeh MC, et al. Functional restoration of elbow flexion in brachial plexus injuries: results in 167 patients (excluding obstetric brachial plexus injury). J Hand Surg Am 1993;18(2):285–91.

26. Giuffre JL, Kakar S, Bishop AT, et al. Current concepts of the treatment of adult brachial plexus injuries. J Hand Surg Am 2010 Apr;35(4):678–88. Erratum in: J Hand Surg Am. 2010 Jul;35(7):1226. Kakar, Sanjiv [corrected to Kakar, Sanjeev]. PMID: 20353866.

27. Bertelli JA. Free Reverse Gracilis Muscle Combined with Steindler Flexorplasty for Elbow Flexion Reconstruction After Failed Primary Repair of Extended Upper-Type Paralysis of the Brachial Plexus. J Hand Surg Am 2019;44(2):112–20.

28. Martins-Filho FVF, do Carmo Iwase F, Silva GB, et al. Do technical components of microanastomoses influence the functional outcome of free gracilis muscle transfer for elbow flexion in traumatic brachial plexus injury? Orthop Traumatol Surg Res 2021;107(2):102827.

29. Nicoson MC, Franco MJ, Tung TH. Donor nerve sources in free functional gracilis muscle transfer for elbow flexion in adult brachial plexus injury. Microsurgery 2017;37(5):377–82.

30. Cho AB, Bersani Silva G, Pisani MJ, et al. Comparison between donor nerves to motorize the free functional gracilis muscle transfer for elbow flexion: Retrospective study of 38 consecutive cases in traumatic adult brachial plexus injuries. Microsurgery 2019;39(5):400–4.

31. Coulet B, Boch C, Boretto J, et al. Free Gracilis muscle transfer to restore elbow flexion in brachial plexus injuries. Orthop Traumatol Surg Res 2011;97(8):785–92.

32. Terzis JK, Kostopoulos VK. Free muscle transfer in posttraumatic plexopathies: part III. The hand. Plast Reconstr Surg 2009;124(4):1225–36.
33. Doi K, Kuwata N, Muramatsu K, et al. Double muscle transfer for upper extremity reconstruction following complete avulsion of the brachial plexus. Hand Clin 1999;15(4):757–67.
34. Maldonado AA, Romero-Brufau S, Kircher RNMF, et al. Free Functioning Gracilis Muscle Transfer for Elbow Flexion Reconstruction after Traumatic Adult Brachial Pan-Plexus Injury: Where Is the Optimal Distal Tendon Attachment for Elbow Flexion? Plast Reconstr Surg 2017;139(1):128–36.
35. Terzis JK, Kostopoulos VK. Free Muscle Transfer in Posttraumatic Plexopathies Part II: The Elbow. Hand (N Y) 2010;5(2):160–70.
36. Doi K, Hattori Y, Ikeda K, et al. Significance of shoulder function in the reconstruction of prehension with double free-muscle transfer after complete paralysis of the brachial plexus. Plast Reconstr Surg 2003;112(6):1596–603.
37. Ballestín A, Malzone G, Menichini G, et al. ASO Visual Abstract: New Robotic System with Wristed Micro-Instruments Allows Precise Reconstructive Microsurgery. Ann Surg Oncol 2023. https://doi.org/10.1245/s10434-023-13632-y.

Functioning Free Muscle Transplantation to Restore Finger Movement for Sequalae of Volkmann Ischemic Contracture

Kota Hayashi, MD, David Chwei-Chin Chuang, MD, Tommy Nai-Jen Chang, MD, Johnny Chuieng-Yi Lu, MD, MSCI*

KEYWORDS

- Volkmann ischemic contracture • Functioning free muscle transplantation • Finger movement

KEY POINTS

- Application of the functioning free muscle transplantation (FFMT) for treatment of Volkmann ischemic contracture (VIC) is markedly different from trauma and brachial plexus injury.
- Joint contractures must be corrected, and fibrotic nonviable muscles must be removed before the implementation of FFMT.
- Three-staged strategy is necessary to achieve optimal outcome with FFMT.
- Gracilis FFMT for VIC needs to include a reliable skin flap paddle in order to facilitate closure in the forearm.

 Video content accompanies this article at http://www.hand.theclinics.com.

HISTORY

The term "Volkmann ischemic contracture" was first noted in 1869 by Richard von Volkmann (1830–1889), but it was not until 1881 that the term was officially coined.[1,2] von Volkmann had observed that tight bandages did not cause paralysis of nerves, but instead caused rapid and significant deterioration of muscle function, leading to limb paralysis and contractures. Animal investigations in 1884 confirmed that the pathologic findings of Volkmann contracture were the result of oxygen deprivation. In 1890, Hildebrand used the term "Volkmann contracture" for the first time. In 1909, Thomas[3] accumulated and analyzed 107 previously reported cases from the available literature.

He confirmed that extrinsic pressure was not the sole cause of Volkmann contracture, as some cases occurred without bandages or splints being applied. In 1911, Bardenheuer described treatment by means of fasciotomy and illustrated the "apo-neurectomy" in the literature. In 1914, Murphy, and in 1926, Jepson[4] attributed posttraumatic contractures to internal pressure and venous obstruction, suggesting splitting of the forearm fascia to decompress the limb to prevent paralysis and contracture. In 1940, Griffiths emphasized arterial injury and reflex spasm of the collateral vessels as the sole source of muscle ischemia, minimizing the role of tight external dressings. In 1956, Seddon[5,6] described the ellipsoid infarct pattern of muscle infarction common in compartment

Department of Plastic and Reconstructive Surgery, Chang Gung Memorial Hospital, Taipei – Linkou, No. 5, Fuxing Street, Guishan District, Taoyuan City 333, Taiwan
* Corresponding author.
E-mail address: cylu122@gmail.com

Hand Clin 40 (2024) 269–281
https://doi.org/10.1016/j.hcl.2023.08.012

syndrome and emphasized the importance of ischemic injury to nerves. The term "compartment syndrome" was first proposed in 1963 by Reszel and colleagues. It was not until 1975 that Holden[7,8] suggested that compartment syndrome was an acute ischemic condition that could lead to contracture if left untreated. In the same year, Matsen[9] proposed a unified concept of compartment syndrome, suggesting that increased tissue pressure was the common denominator of this disease process. Also in 1975, Whitesides and colleagues[10] described tissue pressures as a determinant of the need for fasciotomy.

PATHOPHYSIOLOGY OF VOLKMANN ISCHEMIC CONTRACTURE

Matsen[9] proposed a unified concept of compartment syndrome that involves various mechanisms of vascular compromise, leading to cellular injury.[8,9,11,12] Increased pressures in the fascial compartments of the forearm, hand, or lower extremities can result from limited space owing to outside pressure or an increase in tissue volume within the rigid compartment. This increased pressure causes venous stasis, leading to muscle ischemia and necrosis, transforming into scar tissue. Trauma, in the form of either continued external pressure or direct crush, can cause arterial damage, hematoma, and edema. Local or systemic hypotension can also decrease the arteriovenous gradient and affect blood circulation. Increased capillary permeability owing to ischemia results in edema, further increasing compartmental pressure and compromising the microcirculation of the muscles and nerves, leading to irreversible ischemia. Ischemic muscles degenerate and become fibrotic and contracted through fibroblastic proliferation, whereas nerves may also be compressed or affected by necrosis. The extent of muscle injury depends on the duration of ischemia and the metabolic rate of the tissue. Prolonged ischemia can ultimately lead to liquefactive necrosis of the muscle compartment.

Pathophysiology of Nerve Injuries in Volkmann Ischemic Contracture

The concomitant injury on the regional nerves owing to ischemia and compression is often neglected.[13] Seddon[5,6] proposed that the initial ischemic insult during the acute compartment syndrome results in nerve damage. Tsuge[14] later suggested that mechanical pressure that develops over time as a result of muscle fibrosis can also develop into nerve lesions. Both neural factors compounded by the target muscle injuries gives the nerve an unfavorable environment, thus explaining the low likelihood for spontaneous recovery if VIC is suspected.

The peripheral nerves are composed of myelinated and unmyelinated fibers within fascicles, enveloped by endoneurium and mesoneurium. Blood flow enters the nerve through the mesoneurium after passing through the vasa nervorum. An injury to the mesoneurium leads to nerve adhesion to surrounding tissue. The endoneurium contains capillaries with tight junctions that form the blood-nerve barrier (BNB), which shares similarities with the blood-brain barrier. Compromise of the perfusion can result in BNB breakage, leading to leakage of proteins, lymphocytes, and fibroblasts, causing endoneurial edema, inflammation, and scar formation.[15–18] This leads to demyelination (axonotmesis) in acute ischemia, and axonal loss (neurotmesis) in chronic ischemia.[19] The other aspect of nerve injuries in VIC arises from compression of the regional nerves owing to the fibrotic nature of the scarred tissues in the environment. As such, nerves can be compressed in acute, subacute, or chronic fashion.[19] Powell and Myers[19] evaluated the effects of increased pressures in rat sciatic nerves over intervals of 4 hours up to 28 days, observing edema, inflammation, and fibrin deposits, followed by fibrous tissue proliferation, fibrosis, and infiltration of mast cells and macrophages. Chronic nerve compression models showed a dose-response relationship between compression duration and neural injury.[20–23] Initial changes included a breakdown in the BNB, followed by subperineurial edema, fibrosis, localized and then diffuse demyelination, and finally, Wallerian degeneration with axonal loss. This is one of the reasons that earlier intervention for VIC is indicated in the perspective of nerve ischemia, and not just through the perspective of tendon and muscle contracture.

CLASSIFICATIONS

VIC has been classified according to the severity of the contracture by Seddon[5,6] and also by Tsuge[14] according to muscle group involvement, extent, and function. The classification systems can be useful in guiding functional reconstruction. The most commonly used classification system is that proposed by Tsuge (**Fig. 1**). Established Volkmann contracture was divided into mild, moderate, and severe types, according to the extent of muscle involvement.

Mild

Localized Volkmann contracture usually involves principally the deep flexor compartment (flexor digitorum profundus of long and ring fingers most affected), with little or no nerve involvement.

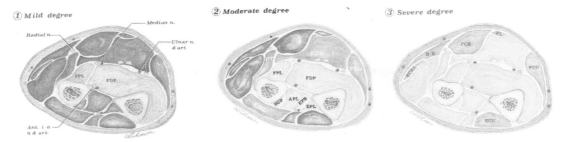

Fig. 1. Severity of VIC depending on the level of muscles involved in the forearm: (1) mild degree, (2) moderate degree, (3) severe degree. The order of muscle involvement is as follows: third layer (FDP, FPL) → second layer (FDS, FCU, PT) → first layer (FCR, PL) → forearm extensors. APL, abductor pollicis longus; art, artery; B-R, brachioradialis; ECRL, extensor carpi radialis longus; ECU extensor carpi ulnaris; EPB, extensor pollicis brevis; FCU, flexor carpi ulnaris; FDS, flexor digitorum superficialis; i.o., interosseous; PL, palmaris longus; PT, pronator teres; SUP, supinator.

Moderate

Most or all of flexor digitorum profundus and flexor pollicis longus are involved, with partial flexor digitorum superficialis. Neurologic impairment is present, with sensory disturbances in the median nerve more than ulnar nerve.

Severe

The entire flexor compartment is involved, with varying involvement of the extensor compartment, with severe median and ulnar neurologic deficits, including sensory deficits and intrinsic dysfunction. The radial nerve may be involved.

The deeper compartments, especially those adjacent to bone, usually have higher interstitial pressures during compartment syndrome. The flexor digitorum profundus and flexor pollicis longus muscles are first affected. In the mild contractures, only a portion of the flexor digitorum profundus undergoes scarring, usually affecting the ring and long fingers. In severe contractures, all 4 digits are involved. The flexor digitorum superficialis and pronator teres (PT) are less often affected. In the most severe cases, however, the digital and wrist flexors and extensors may all be involved. Collateral circulation to the more superficial portions of the forearm muscles helps perfuse the superficial muscles. In the forearm, muscle degeneration commonly occurs in the middle third of the forearm, where the muscle belly is located, with less involvement in the proximal or distal third of the forearm. If the initial signs of compartment syndrome are not picked up and emergent decompression is not performed, after the swelling resolves, the ischemic muscles undergo fibrosis, leading to contracture. A scar band can develop within the muscle or group of muscles.[24]

CLINICAL PICTURE

Patients with limb contractures typically do not have rest pain, but pain initiated by passive manipulation of the joints is a typical sign. Insufficient function of the limb results from severe contracture of the involved muscles, leading to little movement of the tendons and progressive stiffness of the joints. If ischemic neuropathy is also present, paresthesia of the median and/or ulnar distribution may be present, in addition to extrinsic and intrinsic muscle paralysis.

It may take weeks or months for the characteristic deformity of ischemic contracture to manifest. In cases where the forearm and hand are severely affected, the upper limb deformity typically includes protonation of the forearm, flexion of the wrist, thumb, and interphalangeal joint, as well as extension of the digital metacarpophalangeal joint **(Fig. 2)**. The combination of metacarpophalangeal joint extension and proximal interphalangeal joint flexion results in a claw-hand deformity. Although milder contractures may be manually correctable through physiotherapy, persistent muscle imbalance and limited joint movement can ultimately lead to fixed joint deformity. In children, an untreated deformity will progress until skeletal maturity because the ischemic muscles are unable to elongate during growth of the limb. Even when the contractures are treated, the affected extremity is shortened owing to tethering across the physis.[24]

MANAGEMENT
Conservative Treatment

Treatment aims for VIC include striving to restoring sensory and motor function, reducing pain, and reestablishing circulation to affected muscles and nerves.[24-26] The severity of the contracture determines the treatment, with Tsuge and Seddon classifying them accordingly to conservative or surgical treatment. Conservative treatment is typically reserved for mild contractures and involves mobilization and physiotherapy to improve passive joint motion and active muscle force. Methods

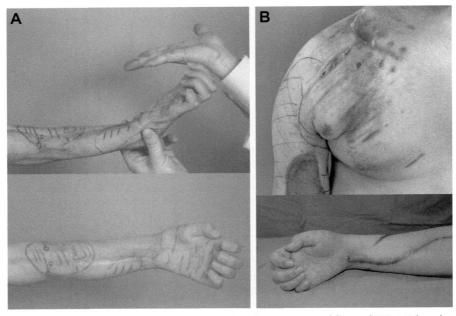

Fig. 2. Characteristic deformity of the hand in VIC. (*A*) Flexed contracture of finger (PIPJ, DIPJ) and wrist, severe tenderness with passive extension, sensory deficit, pronated forearm, intrinsic muscle paralysis, claw fingers, and thumb-in-palm deformity. (*B*) Subclavian artery rupture postarterial bypass. Delayed fasciotomy resulted in flexor contracture of fingers and wrist, with protonation contracture also present. PIPJ, proximal interphalangeal joint; DIPJ, distal interphalangeal joint.

include passive stretching, splinting, serial casting, and wedge application. Initially, the contracture of the wrist is targeted, followed by finger and thumb deformities. In children, splinting is continued until skeletal maturity.

In contrast, moderate and severe contractures require potential staged surgeries and supplementary physiotherapy to maximize outcomes. Moderate and severe contractures are usually recalcitrant to therapy, with limited benefit from stretching and splinting alone.

Operative Treatment

A variety of surgical techniques have been proposed, including bony and soft tissue management. Bone procedures include diaphyseal shortening,[27] arthrodesis,[24] and proximal row carpectomy. Soft tissue procedures include excision of the infarcted muscle, fractional or "Z"-lengthening of the affected muscles, muscle sliding operations (flexor origin muscle slide),[28,29] neurolysis, tendon transfers,[5,6,14] and functioning free muscle transplantation (FFMT), as well as combinations of these procedures. These techniques are selected according to the severity of the contracture. This review focuses on FFMT performed for more severe contractures of the forearm.

Timing of Surgery

The timing of surgery in cases of VIC remains a topic of debate, as there is no clear consensus on the best course of action (**Table 1**).

Seddon and Tsuge[5,6,14] advocated for a delay of at least 3 to 6 months, allowing time for assessment of muscle viability, muscle regeneration, and functional recovery of extensors that might be used as motors for tendon transfers. They thought that nerve damage was due solely to the initial ischemia, and that delay would result in nerve recovery. In contrast, Chuang and colleagues[30] emphasized the benefits of early exploration within 3 weeks of injury or after emergency fasciotomy. Chuang and colleagues found that, in severe VIC, muscle necrosis is extensive and easily distinguished from viable muscle, rendering any possible muscle regeneration insignificant. Early debridement can prevent fibrotic compression responsible for further nerve damage, allowing maximum recovery of intrinsic muscle function and sensory recovery.

Nerve injury in VIC initially occurs as a result of ischemia, but may worsen over time with developing muscle fibrosis. It is a dynamic process that, if left untreated, results in permanent loss of protective sensation and intrinsic function, and sometimes severe pain. Chuang and colleagues' study[30]

Table 1
Comparison between early and late intervention for Volkmann ischemic contracture

	Early Intervention	Late Intervention
Timing	Within 3 wk	At least 3–6 mo
Indication	Severe cases	Well-selected mild cases
Muscle infarct	Muscle necrosis is extensive and easily distinguished from viable muscle, rendering any possible muscle regeneration insignificant	Because of doubts about discerning muscle viability, the possibility of muscle regeneration, and to await any functional recovery of the extensors that might be used as motors for tendon transfers
Nerve injury	Early excision of the infarcted muscles, especially the deep-seated muscles, can reduce nerve compression owing to fibrosis substantially and allow preservation of the intrinsic function of the median and ulnar nerves or at least preservation of some or all of the function of the ulnar nerve	Muscle infarct excision together with neurolysis is difficult. If left untreated, this results in permanent loss of protective sensation and intrinsic function, and sometimes severe pain

demonstrated superior outcomes in restoring sensation and intrinsic function of the hand in patients who underwent early infarct excision. The wait-and-see approach may be acceptable in pediatric populations and a few well-selected adult patients with mild cases. However, for most patients, early intervention is preferred to prevent irreversible damage to nerves and muscles and to optimize the chances of recovery.[13]

History of Functional Free Muscle Transplantation

In 1970, Tamai and colleagues[31] reported successful free rectus femoris muscle transplantation using microneurovascular techniques in dogs. In 1973, surgeons in Shanghai transplanted a portion of the pectoralis major muscle to the forearm.[32] That same year, Harii and colleagues[33] performed the first successful transplantation of a free functioning gracilis muscle for reanimation of facial paralysis. In 1975, Ikuta and colleagues[34] transplanted the free functioning pectoralis major muscle to obtain flexion of the thumb and 4 fingers in a case of severe VIC. Subsequent clinical cases were reported by Schenck[35] and Manktelow and McKee.[36] In 1978, Terzis and colleagues[37] provided the first functional assessment of muscle transplantation in laboratory animals.

Three-Stage Surgical Approach

The authors prefer the three-stage approach (3 Rs) for moderate to severe contractures, which include the following[30,38,39]:

1. REMOVE: Remove questionably viable muscles, scar excision, nerve decompression, neurolysis, nerve reconstruction
2. REHABILITATION: Restore passive range of motion in wrist and fingers
3. REPLACE: Use FFMT to restore finger movement, as well as skin flap replacement for skin deficiency

FFMT may be the only possible reconstructive option following excision of the infarcted muscle. In the acute stage, the immediate application of FFMT without restoring passive range of motion and removing infarcted tissue is unwise. Poor results may ensue owing to the inadequate wound bed and inability to recognize the condition of the recipient nerve. A staged procedure is more appropriate, requiring extensive debridement and nerve exploration, followed by FFMT after at least 6 months of physiotherapy. Aggressive rehabilitation before performing FFMT is especially important to achieve adequate hand function with sensation and movement. If there is bony nonunion, FFMT should be further delayed.

First stage: remove infarct muscle and neurolysis

The first stage of the procedure serves multiple purposes.[5,30] The first stage is to diagnose which muscles and nerves are affected and determine if the extensor tendons are involved. If not, the focus shifts to finger flexion. In cases where extensor tendons are involved, a multistaged double FFMT strategy is recommended, reconstructing the extensors first, followed by the flexors. The procedure also aims to remove all fibrotic or nonviable tissue. The second stage assesses nerve damage and performs neurolysis, as well as evaluates any remaining sensory and intrinsic muscle function. Achieving good hand function in severe upper limb injuries, such as Volkmann contracture, largely depends on the recovery of intrinsic hand function. Last, the procedure prepares the patient for intensive rehabilitation. Joint contractures need to be released intraoperatively and in postoperative rehabilitation. Prompt neurolysis and removal of fibrotic muscles facilitate better nerve recovery, to restore sensation in the hand, and increases the likelihood of intrinsic muscle recovery.

At this stage, the superficial and deep muscles of the forearm are examined for viability (**Fig. 3**). The deeper muscles are more prone to ischemia upon compression. Therefore, initial examination of the forearm muscles, especially in the superficial compartment, can deceive inexperienced surgeons if appearing relatively normal. If the superficial muscles are pale, fibrotic, or show weak or no contraction when the nerve is stimulated, they should be excised to prevent later tendon adhesion in the lower forearm or carpal tunnel. Upon excision, the deep muscles become visible. If the deep flexor muscles are nonviable, they should be removed en bloc up to the junction with healthy muscle (**Fig. 4**). The tendinous portions are preserved for later reconstruction. These tendons are sutured together and fixed to the dermis with a marker suture. Generally, the PT and upper margin of the flexor muscles are healthy and preserved for coverage of neurovascular structures. Determining which muscles to excise or preserve can be tricky in the early stages after compartment syndrome. Extrinsic forearm muscles that appear yellow or pale red with questionable viability should be excised, and a lack of contraction to electric stimulation (with no tourniquet) is an ensuring sign that the muscle will not likely recover. If the exploration is done at a more delayed time point after compartment syndrome, piecemeal removal of fibrotic muscle can be performed. A good rule of thumb is the use of the Finger Test: if the muscle tissue is easily torn or is too fragile or brittle to finger manipulation, it should be removed.

Assessing the nerve The median nerve runs between the superficial and deep flexor compartments of the forearm and is located more centrally, thus making it more liable to ischemia. Severe ischemia may cause the median nerve to narrow significantly, resulting in a grayish-yellow color and avascular region. The nerve swells distal to the compression point and typically does not return to a normal diameter owing to Wallerian degeneration. Immediate decompression with neurolysis can restore sensation in the hand, but thenar function may be compromised after prolonged ischemia. The ulnar nerve on the other hand tends to be less severely affected, and as such, intrinsic musculature of the hand can be preserved. However, if the ulnar nerve's diameter, color, and consistency are abnormal, there is high risk for irreversible recovery.

Blood flow to the nerve is a crucial aspect of nerve assessment. Necrotic muscle excision should be performed under tourniquet control for better evaluation of blood flow. Once the tourniquet is released, external blood flow to the nerve should return. It is essential to carefully evaluate the caliber of the nerve and the presence of bands of Fontana under microscopic dissection. The

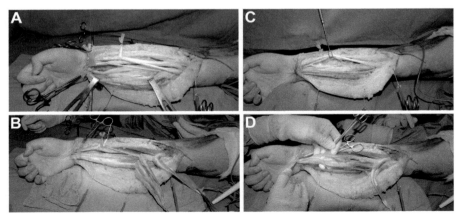

Fig. 3. Right C5-T1 root avulsion brachial plexus injury with concomitant subclavian artery rupture. Patient presented with right forearm contracture, and intraoperative exploration showed extensive VIC of the (*A, B*) superficial and (*C, D*) deep compartments of the flexor muscles.

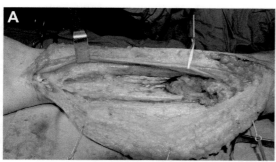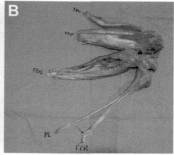

Fig. 4. (*A*) Following excision of flexor muscles of the superficial and deep compartments and neurolysis of median and ulnar nerves. Myomectomy of the pronator quadratus was required to correct protonation contracture. Unhealthy, fibrotic muscles can be peeled off manually using the "Finger test." (*B*) Complete removal of the muscle mass with preservation of the distal tendons in the wrist for future FFMT preparation.

bands of Fontana are reflections of light from axons traveling in a wavy, sinusoidal path, which promote elasticity in peripheral nerves.[40,41] These bands can disappear owing to mechanical stretch or compression injury,[42] but external neurolysis can restore them. In instances where blood flow does not return after the release of long nerve segments from surrounding fibrotic muscles, and the nerve remains pale white,[43] it is important to determine whether this is due to disruption of external blood flow or localized mechanical compression or stricture formation. The latter may benefit from opening the external neural sheath and releasing the stricture. In cases where both circulation and bands of Fontana are absent, opening the thickened perineural sheath is recommended.[12] If notable disruption and thinning are present, resection of the damaged segment followed by replacement with an intercalary nerve graft may be necessary.

In the earlier phase, removal of the infarcted muscle can decompress the nerve. Combined with neurolysis, there is a high possibility to restore intrinsic function in the hand with sensory recovery. Early intervention within the first month of injury can prevent significant thinning or rupture of nerve trunks.[30] In later stages, especially beyond 6 months, neurolysis may not be enough. Loss of intrinsic musculature should be expected and explained to the patient at this stage of the treatment to alleviate the expectations of a fully functional hand.

Second stage: rehabilitation to restore passive range of motion

Physiotherapy plays a crucial role in the surgical treatment of VIC and thus is distinguished as an individual stage of treatment that must be performed before FFMT inset. The primary goals are to (1) restore passive range of motion of all affiliated

joints in the hand and wrist, including release of joint contractures; (2) allow time for spontaneous recovery of sensory and intrinsic musculature after decompression and neurolysis; and (3) ensure viability and function of the remaining muscles if preserved.

Physiotherapy addresses muscle imbalances and stiffness. Therapists use various techniques, such as stretching exercises, joint mobilization, and soft tissue manipulation, to improve flexibility and range of motion in the affected limb. These interventions help to lengthen tight muscles, release scar tissue, and reduce joint stiffness, allowing for improved functional movement. Another crucial aspect of physiotherapy is strengthening the weakened muscles. Through targeted exercises and resistance training, physiotherapists work to rebuild muscle strength and improve muscle endurance. Strengthening exercises also help to prevent further muscle wasting and promote better overall muscle balance. In addition to exercises, physiotherapists may use splinting and bracing techniques. Customized splints or braces can help maintain proper alignment, prevent contractures, and support the affected limb during functional activities. These devices are often used to immobilize specific joints while allowing movement in other joints, facilitating optimal healing and recovery. Physiotherapy may also incorporate pain management strategies. Therapists use various modalities, such as heat therapy, cold therapy, ultrasound, and electrical stimulation, to relieve pain, reduce inflammation, and promote tissue healing. These modalities can provide symptomatic relief, allowing individuals to engage in therapy more comfortably and effectively.

Continued rehabilitation for a minimum of 6 months is required to obtain near full extension in the metacarpophalangeal and interphalangeal joints. Flexion contractures need to be avoided.

If tendon adhesions are present, tenolysis may be added before FFMT. The goal of full passive range of motion cannot be emphasized enough to achieve optimal outcomes with FFMT.

Third stage: replacement of function using functional free muscle transplantation

If the injury involves both flexor and extensor musculature, 2 separate muscles are required to replace both functions, and this would be expanded to a two-staged procedure.[39,44–47] The extensors (extensor digitorum communis [EDC], extensor pollicis longus [EPL]) should be reconstructed first, and the flexors (flexor digitorum profundus [FDP], flexor pollicis longus [FPL]) should be reconstructed in a second stage after the extensors have become innervated. This keeps the extensors one step ahead of the flexors until final rehabilitation is achieved and a plateau is reached at about 1 year. If finger flexion is restored first, the imbalance will make it difficult for extensor rehabilitation.

Functional free muscle transplantation for flexor replacement (FDP, FPL)

1. Preparation of the forearm: The skin on the recipient forearm should be elevated laterally and medially as skin flaps to create space for the transplanted FFMT. It is important to visualize the muscle flap as a space-occupying

lesion when placed inside a tight space like the forearm compartment. This is why debridement of nonviable muscle is important (to create space), why the skin flaps in the recipient forearm must be fully elevated before FFMT inset (to cover the tendons), and why the gracilis muscle should be harvested with an attached skin flap (to facilitate closure). During dissection, scar tissue should be generously removed to create space. Care should be taken not to damage the median and ulnar nerves during dissection, especially when prior neurolysis or reconstruction might have been performed.

Selection of a healthy donor nerve is an important factor in determining success. The proximal motor branches of the median nerve, such as the PT branch, the flexor carpi radialis (FCR) branch, and also the anterior interosseous nerve (AION) are all possible donors to innervate the FFMT. The sensory branch to the hand, and the accompanying thenar branch, must not be violated. The recipient vessels could either be radial or ulnar arteries, and the authors' past experiences have been to perform end-to-end anastomosis to the radial artery without compromise of the circulation of the recipient limb. If there is questionable

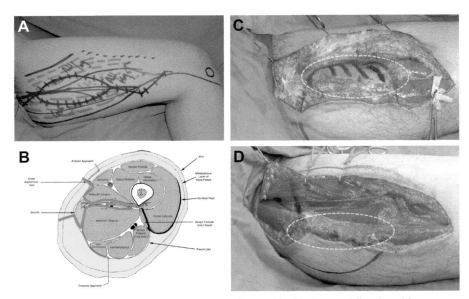

Fig. 5. (*A, B*) Design of the gracilis musculocutaneous flap, with the skin paddle placed between gracilis and adductor muscle, to incorporate the septocutaneous and the proximal myocutaneous perforators. (*C*) Inclusion of the deep fascia of the adductor longus muscle to the skin paddle of the gracilis to ensure that the septum is included. The *circled dashed line* refers to the deep fascia of the adductor longus muscle that should be included within the harvest of the gracilis myocutaneous flap (*D*) The deep fascia of the adductor longus is sutured to the skin paddle to prevent tension on the septocutaneous perforators. The adductor longus should appear exposed without the overlying deep fascia. The *circled dashed line* refers to the deep fascia of the adductor longus muscle that is sutured to the gracilis skin paddle.

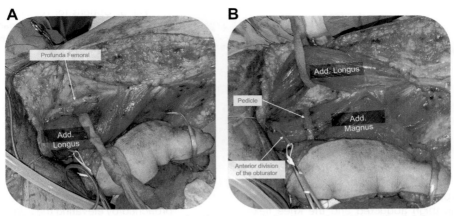

Fig. 6. (*A*) The adductor longus muscle is looped with gauze to help dissect the full length of the vascular pedicle of the gracilis muscle going into the profunda femoris vessels. (*B*) With dissection of the vascular pedicle, the branches to the adductor longus and adductor longus should be ligated. With the adductor longus fully lifted, the anterior division of obturator nerve can be traced proximally all the way to the obturator foramen if length is needed. Add., adductor.

circulation in the forearm, then end-to-side anastomosis to the brachial artery more proximally is another option.

In the distal forearm, the FDP tendons are identified. The FDP tendons are sutured to one another under appropriate tension to mimic the normal finger cascade. The FPL should also be identified. If it is to be incorporated into the single muscle transplant, it should flex slightly after the fingers. In this way, the thumb is not caught in the palm, thus decreasing the effectiveness of the grip. It should flex down after the fingers to provide for thumb-index apposition. The medial humerus periosteum on the distal humerus is prepared as the proximal anchoring site for the gracilis.

2. Harvesting the gracilis muscle: The muscle is harvested simultaneously using the two-team approach. The gracilis is the authors' first choice because of its shape, good excursion, long and single innervated motor nerve, reliably located vascular pedicle, overlying skin flap, and acceptable donor site morbidity. The use of the ipsilateral gracilis facilitates vascular anastomoses when inset into the ipsilateral volar forearm.

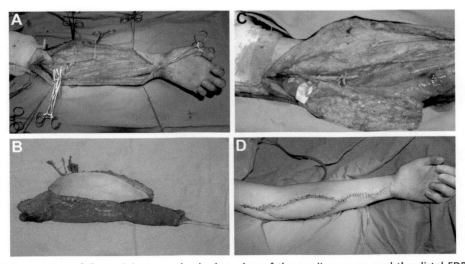

Fig. 7. (*A*) Preparation of the recipient vessels, the branches of the median nerve, and the distal FDP tendons before the FFMT is inset. (*B*) Harvest of the gracilis FFMT (from the ipsilateral thigh). (*C*) Inset of the muscle, with vascular anastomosis and the nerve coaptation performed. (*D*) Closure of the wound, with specific emphasis on the gracilis skin paddle, which can help decrease tension and also provide room to not compress the pedicle anastomosis sites.

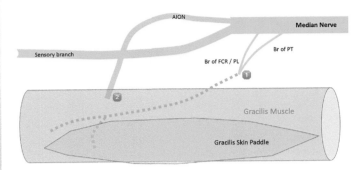

Fig. 8. Options for reinnervation of the FFMT. (1) Nerve-to-nerve coaptation, (2) direct muscle neurotization. Br., branch.

The patient is placed in a supine position with the thigh abducted and the knee flexed. First, skin incisions are placed on proximal and distal parts of the gracilis muscle to identify its location. The skin paddle is designed on the lateral part of the gracilis muscle and the medial part of the adductor longus muscle (**Fig. 5**). Inclusion of the adductor longus deep fascia helps preserve the septum between the adductor longus and gracilis muscles.[39] Fat tissue should be included as little as possible, but care should be taken not to damage the musculocutaneous perforators, especially in the proximal half of the gracilis.[45] It is also important to preserve the deep fascia around the gracilis to maintain perfusion of the distal skin paddle and to prevent adhesions to the surrounding tissue after transplantation.[46,47]

The neurovascular pedicle is then approached by elevating the adductor longus anteriorly (**Fig. 6**). The main vascular pedicle enters the gracilis in 2 or 3 branches, 8 to 12 cm distal to the pubic tubercle. The motor nerve of the gracilis is a branch of the anterior division of the obturator nerve and enters the pedicle just proximal to the vessels at an angle of 45°. The obturator nerve emerges from the obturator foramen under the pectineus muscle and divides into anterior and posterior divisions. The anterior division passes between the adductor longus and brevis, providing motor branches to both muscles before giving the motor branch to the gracilis muscle. The medial cutaneous nerve of the thigh, a branch of the obturator nerve, courses just lateral to the motor nerve of the gracilis on the undersurface of the adductor longus muscle. It is

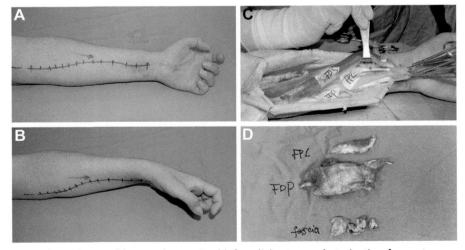

Fig. 9. A greater than 50-year-old man who received left radial artery catheterization for acute coronary artery disease. He developed severe swelling of the forearm immediately after catheterization consistent with compartment syndrome but did not undergo decompression. (*A, B*) He subsequently developed severe flexion contracture with pain in the forearm. (*C*) Exploration showed a healthy superficial compartment but fibrosed deep compartment muscles. (*D*) Removal of FDP and FPL muscles allowed him to passively extend his fingers again.

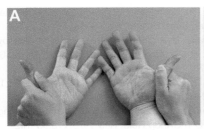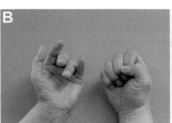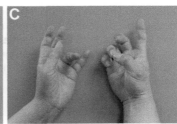

Fig. 10. (*A*) After myomectomy and neurolysis in the first stage, patient is able to reach full extension of the fingers with passive manipulation. (*B*) Weak finger flexion of the DIP joints of the second to fifth fingers is noted. (*C*) Weak opposition of the thumb, in addition to deficiency of thumb IP joint flexion. DIP, distal inter-phalangeal; IP, inter-phalangeal.

important not to confuse the sensory from the motor branches of the obturator nerve by tracing the motor nerve to its entry into the gracilis muscle.

When dissecting the vascular pedicle toward the profunda femoris artery (see **Fig. 6**), branches going upward into the adductor longus must be divided to gain longer length of the pedicle. Often, the paired venae comitantes unite at the takeoff from the profunda femoral vein. The motor nerve to the gracilis is traced as proximal as possible to the obturator foramen, where it is proximally divided. The entire gracilis is elevated from the thigh by detaching its proximal attachment from the pubic ramus, and then cutting the tendinous portion of the gracilis in the thigh. There is technically no need to go all the way to detach the distal tendinous attachment of the gracilis from the medial tibia, because length of the gracilis muscle is typically not an issue when inset into the forearm. Once the forearm dissection is completed and ready to receive the transplanted muscle, the vascular pedicle should be divided. In this way, the muscle ischemia time can be minimized (preferably within 1 hour).

3. Gracilis muscle transplantation to the forearm (**Fig. 7**): The gracilis muscle is securely fixed to the medial humerus periosteum, and the vessels are repaired to minimize ischemia time. Either end-to-end or end-to-side anastomosis to the recipient artery is acceptable, but care should be taken to avoid redundant vessels after anastomoses. The site of tendon repair is marked on the FDP, and the distal tendon repair is performed by weaving the gracilis tendon into the FDP tendons in maximum tension. The nerve repair should be done as close to the gracilis muscle as possible to minimize reinnervation time. In cases where the deep

and superficial muscles of the entire flexor compartment are removed, the proximal motor branches (PT, FCR) of the median nerve are coapted directly to the obturator nerve of the gracilis, whereas the more distal branches (FDS, AION) can be plugged into the muscle tissue directly (**Fig. 8**). If only the deep flexor muscles are absent after the first stage, the AION will likely be the choice of donor nerve for the FFMT.

4. Postoperative care: The extremity is immobilized with a long arm splint after the skin has been closed. It is preferable to have the elbow at 70° to 90° flexion and the wrist slightly flexed to take the tension off the origin and insertion of the muscle. The finger metacarpophalangeal joints should be maintained in a flexed position of 90°, and the thumb should be abducted with the interphalangeal joint slightly flexed.

Case demonstration is shown in **Figs. 9** and **10** and Video 1.

Functional free muscle transplantation for extensor (EDC, EPL) For EDC replacement, the transferred muscle-end fixation point is the lateral epicondyle of the humerus proximally and the 4 conjoined tendons of the EDC distally. Regarding the recipient nerve, the posterior interosseous nerve is commonly used. Attention should be given to preservation of the superficial radial nerve, the ECRB branch, and the supinator branch if these proximal structures are still functional. Harvesting the contralateral gracilis muscle for extensor reconstruction allows easier access to the vascular anastomoses on the extensor side, while using the radial artery as the recipient artery.

SUMMARY

VIC is a devastating condition that affects multiple tissues, including muscles, nerves, skin, and joints. Recognition of the degree of injury to different tissues involved is critical to restoring functional outcome. This requires a staged approach that focuses on achieving maximum range of motion. FFMT can restore finger movement in a paralyzed limb but requires a three-staged approach to maximize the benefits of FFMT, leading to meaningful finger extrinsic function.

CLINICS CARE POINTS

- Application of the functioning free muscle transplantation in Volkmann ischemic contracture is markedly different from trauma and brachial plexus injury.
- Joint contractures must be corrected, and fibrotic nonviable muscles must be removed before the implementation of functioning free muscle transplantation.
- Nerve injury is an often neglected in Volkmann ischemic contracture. This potentially has a component of both compression neuropathy and traumatic avulsion injury, thus making it extremely difficult to manage.
- Restoring passive and active range of motion is key to maximizing functional outcome,
- Three-staged strategy is recommended, with functioning free muscle transplantation as the final stage.
- Gracilis functioning free muscle transplantation for Volkmann ischemic contracture needs to include a reliable skin flap paddle in order to facilitate closure in the forearm.

DISCLOSURE

The authors have no financial interest to declare in relation to the content of this article. No funding was received for this article.

SUPPLEMENTARY DATA

Supplementary data related to this article can be found online at https://doi.org/10.1016/j.hcl.2023.08.012.

REFERENCES

1. Trice M, Colwell CW. A historical review of compartment syndrome and Volkmann's ischemic contracture. Hand Clin 1998;14:335–41.
2. Volkmann R. Ischaemic muscle paralyses and contractures. J Hand Surg Br 2005;30:233–4.
3. Thomas JJ III. Nerve Involvement in the Ischaemic Paralysis and Contracture of Volkmann. Ann Surg 1909;49:330–70.
4. Jepson PN. Ischaemic contracture: experimental study. Ann Surg 1926;84(6):785–95.
5. Seddon HJ. Volkmann's contracture: treatment by excision of the infarct. J Bone Joint Surg Br 1956;38:152–74.
6. Seddon H. Volkmann's Ischaemia. Br Med J 1964;1:1587–92.
7. Holden CE. Compartmental syndromes following trauma. Clin Orthop Relat Res 1975;113:95–102.
8. Holden CE. The pathology and prevention of Volkmann's ischaemic contracture. J Bone Joint Surg Br 1979;61:296–300.
9. Matsen FA 3rd. Compartment syndrome. An unified concept. Clin Orthop Relat Res 1975.
10. Whitesides TE, Haney TC, Morimoto K, et al. Tissue pressure measurements as a determinant for the need of fasciotomy. Clin Orthop Relat Res 1975;113:43–51.
11. Mubarak SJ, Carroll NC. Volkmann's contracture in children: aetiology and prevention. J Bone Joint Surg Br 1979;61:285–93.
12. Gülgönen A. Invited review article: surgery for Volkmann's ischaemic contracture. J Hand Surg Br 2001;26:283–96.
13. Ozer K. Nerve Lesions in Volkmann Ischemic Contracture. J Hand Surg Am 2020;45:746–57.
14. Tsuge K. Treatment of established Volkmann's contracture. J Bone Joint Surg Am 1975;57:925–9.
15. Runkle EA, Mu D. Tight junction proteins: from barrier to tumorigenesis. Cancer Lett 2013;337:41–8.
16. Lim TKY, Shi XQ, Martin HC, et al. Blood-nerve barrier dysfunction contributes to the generation of neuropathic pain and allows targeting of injured nerves for pain relief. Pain 2014;155:954–67.
17. Richner M, Bjerrum OJ, Nykjaer A, et al. The spared nerve injury (SNI) model of induced mechanical allodynia in mice. J Vis Exp 2011;3092.
18. Rempel D, Dahlin L, Lundborg G. Pathophysiology of nerve compression syndromes: response of peripheral nerves to loading. J Bone Joint Surg Am 1999;81:1600–10.
19. Powell HC, Myers RR. Pathology of experimental nerve compression. Lab Invest 1986;55:91–100.
20. Mackinnon SE, Dellon AL, Hudson AR, et al. A primate model for chronic nerve compression. J Reconstr Microsurg 1985;1:185–95.
21. Mackinnon SE, O'Brien JP, Dellon AL, et al. An assessment of the effects of internal neurolysis on a chronically compressed rat sciatic nerve. Plast Reconstr Surg 1988;81:251–8.
22. O'Brien JP, Mackinnon SE, MacLean AR, et al. A model of chronic nerve compression in the rat. Ann Plast Surg 1987;19:430–5.
23. Mackinnon SE, Dellon AL. Evaluation of microsurgical internal neurolysis in a primate median nerve model of chronic nerve compression. J Hand Surg Am 1988;13:345–51.

24. Botte MJ, Keenan MA, Gelberman RH. Volkmann's ischemic contracture of the upper extremity. Hand Clin 1998;14:483–97, x.

25. Sundararaj GD, Mani K. Management of Volkmann's ischaemic contracture of the upper limb. J Hand Surg Br 1985;10:401–3.

26. Pettitt DA, McArthur P. Clinical review: Volkmann's ischaemic contracture. Eur J Trauma Emerg Surg 2012;38:129–37.

27. Domanasiewicz A, Jabłecki J, Kocieba R, et al. Modified Colzi method in the management of established Volkmann contracture–the experience of Trzebnica Limb Replantation Center (preliminary report). Ortop Traumatol Rehabil 2008;10:12–25.

28. Page C. An operation for the relief of flexion-contracture in the forearm. J Bone Joint Surg Am 1923;3:233–4.

29. Sharma P, Swamy MK. Results of the Max Page muscle sliding operation for the treatment of Volkmann's ischemic contracture of the forearm. J Orthop Traumatol 2012;13:189–96.

30. Chuang DC, Carver N, Wei FC. A new strategy to prevent the sequelae of severe Volkmann's ischemia. Plast Reconstr Surg 1996;98:1023–31. discussion 1032-3.

31. Tamai S, Komatsu S, Sakamoto H, et al. Free muscle transplants in dogs, with microsurgical neurovascular anastomoses. Plast Reconstr Surg 1970;46:219–25.

32. Shanghai Sixth People's Hospital. Free muscle transplantation by microsurgical neurovascular anastomoses. Report of a case. Chin Med J (Engl) 1976;2(1):47–50.

33. Harii K, Ohmori K, Torii S. Free gracilis muscle transplantation, with microneurovascular anastomoses for the treatment of facial paralysis. A preliminary report. Plast Reconstr Surg 1976;57:133–43.

34. Ikuta Y, Kubo T, Tsuge K. Free muscle transplantation by microsurgical technique to treat severe Volkmann's contracture. Plast Reconstr Surg 1976;58:407–11.

35. Schenck RR. Free muscle and composite skin transplantation by microneurovascular anastomoses. Orthop Clin North Am 1977;8:367–75.

36. Manktelow RT, McKee NH. Free muscle transplantation to provide active finger flexion. J Hand Surg Am 1978;3:416–26.

37. Terzis JK, Sweet RC, Dykes RW, et al. Recovery of function in free muscle transplants using microneurovascular anastomoses. J Hand Surg Am 1978;3:37–59.

38. Chuang DC, Strauch RJ, Wei FC. Technical considerations in two-stage functioning free muscle transplantation reconstruction of both flexor and extensor functions of the forearm. Microsurgery 1994;15:338–43.

39. Chuang DC. Functioning free-muscle transplantation for the upper extremity. Hand Clin 1997;13:279–89.

40. Merolli A, Mingarelli L, Rocchi L. A more detailed mechanism to explain the "bands of Fontana" in peripheral nerves. Muscle Nerve.;46:540-547.

41. Alvey LM, Jones JFX, Tobin-O'Brien C, et al. Bands of Fontana are caused exclusively by the sinusoidal path of axons in peripheral nerves and predict axon path; evidence from rodent nerves and physical models. J Anat 2019;234:165–78.

42. Mackinnon SE. Pathophysiology of nerve compression. Hand Clin 2002;18:231–41.

43. Jung J, Hahn P, Choi B, et al. Early Surgical Decompression Restores Neurovascular Blood Flow and Ischemic Parameters in an in Vivo Animal Model of Nerve Compression Injury. J Bone Joint Surg Am 2014;96:897–906.

44. Zuker RM, Manktelow RT. Functioning free muscle transfers. Hand Clin 2007;23:57–72.

45. Peek A, Müller M, Ackermann G, et al. The free gracilis perforator flap: anatomical study and clinical refinements of a new perforator flap. Plast Reconstr Surg 2009;123(2):578–88.

46. Addosooki AI, Doi K, Hattori Y. Technique of harvesting the gracilis for free functioning muscle transplantation. Tech Hand Up Extrem Surg 2006;10:245–51.

47. Chidester JR, Leland HA, Navo P, et al. Redefining the Anatomic Boundaries for Safe Dissection of the Skin Paddle in a Gracilis Myofasciocutaneous Free Flap: An Indocyanine Green Cadaveric Injection Study. Plast Reconstr Surg Glob Open 2018;6:e1994.

Surgical Treatment of Lymphedema in the Upper Extremity

Zhi Yang Ng, MBChB, MRCS, PgDip, PhD[a], Xavier Chalhoub, MBBS, BSc, MRCS[b],
Dominic Furniss, DM, MA, MBBCh, FRCS(Plast)[c],*

KEYWORDS

- Upper extremity • Lymphedema • Lymphaticovenous anastomosis • Lymph node transfer

KEY POINTS

- The main physiologic approaches in lymphedema surgery are lymphaticovenous anastomosis (LVA) and vascularized lymph node transfers (LNTs). LVA requires supermicrosurgical techniques and expertise.
- In the appropriately selected patient, LVA alone can improve the patient's quality of life and reduce the affected upper limb volume.
- The mechanism of action and optimal timing of LNTs remain poorly understood. The complexity of LNT surgery is also greater than LVA, so comparative studies demonstrating significant benefit are required before the optimal surgical strategy can be recommended.

 Video content accompanies this article at http://www.hand.theclinics.com.

INTRODUCTION
History, Background, and Definitions

The surgical management of lymphedema was limited historically to debulking approaches such as the Charles procedure and the modified Charles procedures. The latter includes the intervening use of negative pressure dressing after radical excision of lymphedematous tissues, followed by skin grafting 5 to 7 days later. Both procedures result in significant morbidity and cosmetic deformity, due to the loss of fascia and need for skin grafting.[1]

This has since been supplanted by a reductive approach consisting of liposuction, although with the caveat of obligatory lifelong use of compression garments for 23 hours a day postoperatively to minimize the risk of recurrence.[2]

In high-income countries, upper limb lymphedema typically develops secondarily following oncological treatment in the form of ablative lymph node surgery (eg, sentinel lymph node biopsy and axillary clearance) and/or radiotherapy to the involved lymph node basin. This leads to anatomic disruption of the lymphatic system, resulting in the accumulation of protein-rich interstitial fluid, persistent swelling, and eventually, fibro-adipose hypertrophy. Upper limb lymphedema has a negative effect on quality of life, including physical and psychological dysfunction. Furthermore, patients may suffer from recurrent bouts of cellulitis requiring antibiotics and hospital admission.

[a] Department of Plastic and Reconstructive Surgery, John Radcliffe Hospital, Oxford University Hospitals NHS Foundation Trust, Headley Way, Headington, Oxford, OX3 9DU, United Kingdom; [b] Department of Plastic and Reconstructive Surgery, The Royal Free Hospital, Royal Free London NHS Foundation Trust, Pond Street, London, NW3 2QG, United Kingdom; [c] Department of Plastic and Reconstructive Surgery, Nuffield Orthopaedic Centre, Oxford University Hospitals NHS Foundation Trust, Windmill Road, Oxford, OX3 7LD, United Kingdom
* Corresponding author. Nuffield Department of Orthopaedics, Rheumatology, and Musculoskeletal Sciences, University of Oxford.
E-mail address: dominic.furniss@ndorms.ox.ac.uk

Hand Clin 40 (2024) 283–290
https://doi.org/10.1016/j.hcl.2023.10.005
0749-0712/24/© 2023 Elsevier Inc. All rights reserved.

The concept of lymphaticovenous anastomosis (LVA) to bypass the disrupted lymphatic channels was first demonstrated by O'Brien[3] and later, popularized by Koshima through the use of super-microsurgical techniques.[4] Lymph node transfer (LNT) is another procedure following the physiologic approach in the treatment of lymphedema. Essentially, LNT is theorized as a "pump" action whereby excess interstitial fluid is channeled toward the transferred node(s) itself, as well as the induction of lymphangiogenesis to restore normal lymphatic channels.[5]

Unlike other high-income countries such as the United States and Sweden, which now have insurance coverage for the surgical treatment of lymphedema,[6] the United Kingdom's National Health Service does not currently fund such procedures[7] outside of a research setting due to low-certainty evidence.[8] Furthermore, the latest British Lymphology Society guidelines do not make any recommendations about LVA or LNT other than such procedures are possibly beneficial in reducing the frequency of cellulitis in carefully selected patients.[9] Therefore, in the United Kingdom, the mainstay of treatment of lymphedema remains nonsurgical in the form of complete decongestive therapy, or one or more of its individual components that is, manual lymphatic drainage, skin care, compression, and remedial exercises.[10]

Current Evidence

For hand and microsurgeons, the surgical concept of reconstructing the lymphatic system through either LVA or LNT is sound and in line with our training. However, the biology of lymphedema is inherently complex and remains poorly understood. To illustrate, although the focus of the current article is on LVA and LNT, multiple institutions around the world have investigated and reported preliminary results from various combinations of treatment involving the physiologic (LVA and LNT), reductive (liposuction), and debulking (Charles procedure) approaches, when neither LVA or LNT alone was adequate.[11]

The reported clinical efficacy of LVA and LNT is highly variable, with long-term limb volume reduction ranging from 2.4% to 69% and 7.1% to 75%, respectively.[12] Reasons for this wide-ranging discrepancy may include variation in staging systems (MD Anderson, International Society of Lymphology [ISL] and so forth[11]; **Table 1**), measurement methodology (eg, tape vs perometer),[13] and study design (retrospective case series, patient loss to follow-up, exclusion of nonrandomized controlled trials, and so forth) leading to an overall weak evidence base.[8]

Although there have been systematic reviews to further evaluate the accruing evidence, these efforts were undermined by the lack of stringent and robust methodology, including nonadherence to standard reporting guidelines[14] and the inclusion of nonrandomized data.[15] It is therefore no surprise that there remains a paucity of evidence-based clinical guidelines and disconnect in recommendations among different specialties involved in the care of patients with lymphedema.[16] In the ensuing discussion, we shall highlight some practical aspects of lymphedema surgery based on the senior author's experience of more than 10 years.

DISCUSSION
Evaluation, Approach, and Imaging

The initial assessment of all patients includes a thorough history, physical examination focused especially on signs and complications of lymphedema, and limb volume measurements taken with a perometer. All patients, regardless of primary or secondary lymphedema, are evaluated with indocyanine green (ICG) lymphography. For patients who are at high risk of developing secondary upper limb lymphedema, screening with ICG lymphography is usually performed 3 months following completion of cancer treatment (typically for breast cancer) to determine whether lymphedema has started to develop. Further, repeat ICG lymphography screening is then performed at 6-monthly intervals for up to 3 years following cancer treatment.

In patients with established lymphedema, ICG lymphography will determine if they are likely to be a good candidate for surgery (**Fig. 1**A–D). We consider patients to have adequate lymphatic

Table 1 International Society of Lymphology lymphedema staging	
Stage	Symptoms/Clinical Findings
0	Subclinical lymphedema without edema but with evidence of impaired lymphatic function. Can exist for months or years before overt edema develops
I	Reversible pitting edema. Fibrosis not palpable
II	A: Pitting edema not reducible by elevation B: Nonpitting edema secondary to pronounced fibrosis
III	Lymphostatic elephantiasis with progressive fibrosis, acanthosis, hyperkeratosis, and papillomatosis

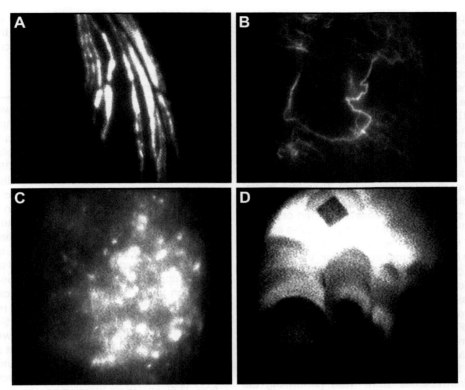

Fig. 1. ICG lymphangiography images showing (*A*) linear, (*B*) splash, (*C*) stardust, and (*D*) diffuse patterns. Different patterns of ICG can be used to grade lymphedema severity. Linear patterns are normal, whereas splash, stardust, and diffuse patterns reflect increasing levels of lymphatic vessel fibrosis and lymphedema severity.

reserve for reconstructive microsurgery whose lymphatics transport ICG dye to the upper arm within a 30-minute timeframe. In general, the sooner patients can access physiologic reconstruction, the greater the remaining function within the lymphatic system, and the better the results of reconstructive microsurgery. However, some patients with longstanding lymphedema may have adequately retained function and can still benefit from surgery. ICG lymphography is also used on the day of surgery to locate functional lymphatics for LVA. We also use ultrasound scanning to locate veins that are close to functional lymphatics, enabling a highly targeted operation as described below.

One of the main confounding factors in lymphedema surgery outcomes is the variation in methodology reported in the literature to assess limb volume. Most commonly, this is done with tape measure, which is subject to high interobserver and intraobserver variability. In particular, results are affected by how "tight" one pulls on the tape and by the distance proximally from the wrist where the first measurement is taken. To mitigate this bias, we use perometry, a technique that applies infrared light and sensors to generate a 3-D

representation of the limb and measure overall limb volume. This was previously demonstrated to be superior to tape measurements for interobserver reliability.[13]

The effects of lymphedema on quality of life are evaluated using the Lymphedema Quality of Life Questionnaire (LYMQOL).[17] This is a validated tool used to assess the domains of function, appearance, symptoms, mood, and overall quality of life in lymphedema patients. We use the LYMQOL preoperatively and at 3, 6, and 12 months postoperatively.[18]

Surgical Technique

Immediate preoperative planning with ICG lymphography and ultrasonography is imperative for surgical planning. First, 25 mg ICG is dissolved in 5 mL of water for injection, and 0.1 mL of this solution is injected using a 30G syringe into the third webspace of the hand, and radial and ulnar borders of the wrist, after an injection of local anesthesia without adrenaline. Gentle massage facilitates ICG uptake, and over around 20 minutes, suitable lymphatic vessels are mapped with the aid of a near infrared camera system and marked on the skin. Typically, as many potential sites for LVA as possible are marked along the length of the upper limb, usually with one in the upper medial arm and 3 in the forearm (**Fig. 2**).

Two consultant microsurgeons will then operate simultaneously to optimize theater efficiency. Patent blue V dye is injected just distal to each planned incision to facilitate lymphatic vessel identification during dissection. Transverse incisions of approximately 2 to 5 cm are then made in the previously marked sites. It should be noted that the superficial lymphatic system closely follows that of the superficial venous system. Therefore, meticulous dissection helps identify the lymphatic vessels should ICG be contraindicated or unsuccessful.[19] Under high magnification, LVAs are performed with 11/0 nylon for vessels that are typically 0.3 to 0.8 mm in diameter. Various anastomotic configurations are deployed depending on anatomic configuration, including end-to-end, end-to-side, side-to-side, and sleeve, the technicalities of which are beyond the scope of this article (**Fig. 3**).[20] We deliberately choose veins with competent valves to avoid venous back flow and anastomotic thrombosis. For small lymphatics, the use of a 4/0 Prolene suture as a temporary intravascular stent while performing the anastomosis greatly facilitates successful microsurgery.[21] Anastomotic patency is then confirmed by observing for passage of lymphatic fluid into the venule (Video 1). This may be delayed by several minutes due to the underlying disease process but can be facilitated with gentle massage distal to the incision. On average, each surgery lasts for about 4 hours.

Postoperative Management

From days 0 to 7, no compression is applied to avoid pressure over the anastomosis and obstructing flow. The limb is elevated and light massage begins distally, progressing toward the incisions. From days 7 to 14, old compression garments are worn while massage and elevation are continued. At day 14, the wounds are examined and sutures removed if needed. At this point, compression can resume as normal along with a gradual return to normal activities.

Clinical Outcomes

In a prospective cohort of 37 patients with breast cancer with unilateral upper limb lymphedema, we have demonstrated (1) reduction in limb volume in 78% of patients at a median follow-up of 6.5 months (range, 3–33 months); (2) in 35% of patients, they were able to completely discontinue compression garments; and (3) 86% of patients reported a better quality of life based on improvement in LYMQOL scores.[18] Of note, results differed between patients with an initial excess volume of more than 5%, 5% to 20%, and more than 20% (difference between affected and unaffected upper limb, as measured by perometry). Although those with a larger initial excess were more likely to show measurable volume reduction, 6 out of 9 patients with less than 5% volume excess were able to discontinue wearing a compression sleeve, compared to 7 out of 18 patients with volume excess 5% to 20% and 0 out of 10 patients with volume excess greater than 20%.[18] Finally, there were no postoperative complications such as persistent lymphatic leak, wound infection, or cellulitis in this group of patients.

Controversies

Lymphaticovenous anastomosis or lymph node transfer?

In the microsurgical lymphedema field, there is debate as to whether LVA or LNT is the best reconstructive option for patients with early-stage lymphedema. It was previously speculated that LNT

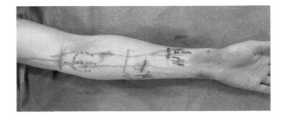

Fig. 3. Lymphatic channels identified preoperatively (*red lines*) with ICG lymphography. Three transverse incisions were subsequently used under a local anesthetic in the left forearm to perform 9 lymphaticovenous anastomoses: 3 proximal (1 sleeve, 2 end-to-end), 3 middle (3 sleeve), and 3 distal (3 sleeve). Note the blue staining of the skin, which is from the use of patent blue intraoperatively to more easily visualize the lymphatic channels identified preoperatively.

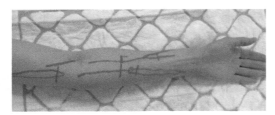

Fig. 2. ICG lymphography performed preoperatively on the day of surgery to locate functional lymphatics for lymphaticovenular anastomosis (as demonstrated by the red markings).

might be more effective than LVA, although 22% of patients required further excisional procedures.[22] However, LVA is a simple procedure performed under local anesthesia as a day case, with a very low risk of complications. In contrast, LNT is a free flap procedure, performed under general anesthesia with associated hospital stay and a far higher risk of complications. Indeed, the overall rate of complications approaches 1 in 4 for LNT and includes hematoma, flap compromise requiring take backs, flap necrosis and loss, lymphorrhea, seroma, and not least, the risk of developing lymphedema at the donor site from iatrogenic damage when harvesting lymph nodes.[23] Therefore, given this risk–benefit ratio, LVA is favored over LNT for early stage disease. Recent evidence, however, suggests that, actually, with advances in imaging technologies (eg, duplex ultrasound and magnetic resonance lymphangiography), functional lymphatics can still be identified even in later stage disease. As such, even in patients with advanced lymphedema, LVAs can still be performed and achieve clinical improvement.[24]

Lymphaticovenous anastomosis number and patency

Although it is intuitive that the greater the number of LVAs performed the greater the likelihood of clinical improvement, clinical evidence suggests that this may be more an issue of quality over quantity. Koshima and colleagues described an average of 4 LVAs for upper extremity lymphedema, and up to 10 when the anatomy was favorable,[4] whereas Mihara and colleagues reported an average of 9.8 LVAs in lower extremity lymphedema compared to 7.0 in controls and arrived at the same conclusion.[25] A single anastomosis has been shown to be effective in lower limb lymphedema.[26] The long-term patency of LVA is difficult to study however. Currently, this is based on visual assessment of ICG lymphography postoperatively, where flow across the anastomosis was considered essentially as "yes" or "no." Unsurprisingly, this leads to highly subjective results—only 30% remained patent at 6 months in one study,[27] whereas another reported at least one LVA remained patent at 12 months in 76% of patients.[28]

Clinical outcomes in terms of decrease in arm circumference, improvement in quality of life, discontinuation of compression garment usage, and decreased frequency of cellulitis episodes were either not reported or did not achieve statistical significance.[28] There are a multitude of possible confounding factors such as surgeon experience, patient compliance, anastomotic technique, and so forth. With improved survival after cancer treatment, the number of patients living with lymphedema is expected to increase and correspondingly, the clinical and financial interest in performing lymphedema surgery has grown exponentially. Unfortunately, there remains much debate in the accepted concepts of lymphedema between institutions, and therefore, training of techniques and approaches despite the ever-increasing number of fellowships in this subject area.[29]

Increasing experience in this field has also revealed that the quality of the remnant, native lymphatic vessels (ie, normal, ectatic, contracted, and sclerotic), and thus, functionality is likely to be important especially with preservation of the smooth muscle component to retain peristaltic movements.[30] Anastomosing severely sclerotic lymphatic vessels, for instance, will lead to minimal therapeutic effects. Therefore, the identification of lymphatic vessels that are still functional is imperative in LVA. Currently, ICG lymphangiography cannot visualize lymphatic flow that is masked beneath dermal back flow patterns[31] and conventional high-frequency ultrasound has been reported to be a useful alternative, even in limbs severely affected by lymphedema.[32] Such conventional high-frequency ultrasound systems are highly operator dependent, however, and cannot distinguish lymphatic vessels smaller than 0.3 mm from subcutaneous veins or nerves.[31] Ultrahigh-frequency ultrasound systems have recently been developed and reports suggest a sensitivity and specificity for the detection of lymphatic vessels (smaller than 0.3 mm) at 94.9% and 98.3%, respectively, compared to 66.3% and 91.3%, respectively, in conventional high-frequency ultrasound.[33] Indeed, ultrahigh-frequency ultrasound assessment of lymphatics correlates with their histologic features[34] that may, therefore, reduce the need for multiple LVAs as described previously.

Prophylactic lymphaticovenous anastomosis surgery or screening?

There is an increasing interest in performing LVAs prophylactically, at the time of axillary dissection for breast cancer. This interest is driven by the increasing incidence of breast cancer, improved survival, and hence, likelihood of increased prevalence of breast cancer-related lymphedema [BCRL] in patients. Hence, the lymphatic microsurgical preventive healing approach (LYMPHA) has been conceived and is increasing in popularity in recent years to prophylactically prevent the development of upper limb BCRL in patients.[35] Again, although appealing in concept, statistics on the incidence of BCRL vary widely but approximate to 30%, which means that 70% of patients would be receiving unnecessary surgery.[36] Unfortunately, we are currently unable to predict which of these patients will go on to develop BCRL postoperatively but, in any case, not every patient with BCRL would require surgical intervention such as LVA.[37] Thus far, studies on the efficacy of LYMPHA as surgical prophylaxis against BCRL, despite promising results, have been limited by short-term follow-up. Indeed, a recent study has shown that with longer term follow-up of more than 4 years, the incidence of BCRL between the LYMPHA and non-LYMPHA groups was no different (31.1% vs 33.3%).[38] Conversely, an earlier, single-center study with similar follow-up of more than 4 years found that BCRL only developed in 4% of patients.[35] Further studies are therefore required to determine the place of prophylactic LVA in the setting of axillary node dissection for breast cancer before widespread adoption. We screen patients at risk of developing lymphedema using ICG lymphography and only intervene when there is evidence of lymphatic dysfunction, which may or may not be symptomatic (ISL stage 0 or 1).

FUTURE DIRECTIONS

In recent years, alternatives to ICG lymphography have been reported in the form of ultrahigh-frequency and high-frequency ultrasound in combination with magnetic resonance lymphangiography to identify functioning lymphatic vessels in patients with more advanced lymphedema.[24] The paradigm that LVA can only be used for ISL Stage I-II lymphedema has been challenged with promising reports of success in patients with more advanced lower limb lymphedema.[39] We anticipate that similar outcomes for upper limb lymphedema will soon be reported.

There has recently been the development of an intriguing concept—vascularized lymph vessel transplant (VLVT).[40] Briefly, this technique does not require any lymphatic microsurgery. Rather, it builds on our existing armamentarium by raising flaps that we are comfortable and familiar with (eg, Superficial Circumflex Iliac Artery Perforator flap [SCIP] and Thoracodorsal Artery Perforator flap [TDAP]) but at the suprafascial level instead captures superficial lymphatic vessels, followed by standard vascular anastomosis. In so doing, the aforementioned risks of LNT can be avoided, and the need for supermicrosurgical expertise and equipment for LVA can also be negated. Most importantly, VLVT is proposed to induce lymphangiogenesis in vivo by respecting the biology of the lymphedema process through what may be a truly physiologic procedure—by insetting

and orienting the flaps (and transferred superficial lymphatics) in line with the native lymphatic vessels at the recipient site.[41]

Finally, the cost-effectiveness of lymphatic reconstruction must be considered. This remains unknown and insurance coverage is not universal among different health-care systems.[42] Nevertheless, mathematical modeling suggests that lifetime decongestive therapy in a theoretic, Stage II breast cancer survivor with BCRL would cost in excess of US$30,000, whereas successful LVA with consequent discontinuation of compression would cost approximately US$15,000.[42] This was further corroborated by a recent study that reported the average cost of surgery (either LVA or LNT) to be around US$11,000.[43]

SUMMARY

Patients with lymphedema are faced with a daily physical and psychological reminder of their previous cancer. In turn, this has financial implications that result from the associated complications such as cellulitis, which necessitate time off work, especially if hospitalization is required. To illustrate, in patients with BCRL, they are faced with up to 12% higher total out-of-pocket costs when excluding productivity losses, and up to 19% higher total out-of-pocket costs when including productivity losses, compared to those without lymphedema.[44]

Although LVA and LNT remain the current mainstay of surgical management, there has been much discrepancy in outcomes between studies and institutions. In the senior author's practice, screening for lymphedema, followed by LVA for early-stage disease, or later stage disease with functioning lymphatic channels is the mainstay of reconstructive treatment, balancing efficacy with a low surgical risk profile. Late-stage disease with fatty accumulation and severely reduced lymphatic function is treated by liposuction and controlled compression therapy. This allows tailored, pathology-driven treatment that is individualized to the patient.

CLINICS CARE POINTS

- LVA alone can improve the ILS stage I-II lymphedema patient's quality of life and reduce the affected upper limb volume.
- LNT remains poorly understood and is associated with higher morbidity, and in our experience, it does not currently confer any benefit over LVA.

- Further studies are required to determine the relative indications for LVA and LNT, the utility of novel developments such as VLVT, and the role of imaging such as high and ultrahigh-frequency ultrasound in altering currently accepted treatment protocols.

DISCLOSURE

D Furniss performs lymphedema surgery as codirector of the Oxford Lymphoedema Practice (https://olp.surgery/) at the Manor Hospital, Oxford, United Kingdom. Z Y. Ng and X Chalhoub have nothing to disclose.

SUPPLEMENTARY DATA

Supplementary data related to this article can be found online at .https://doi.org/10.1016/j.hcl. 2023.10.005

REFERENCES

1. Hassan K, Chang DW. The Charles procedure as part of the modern armamentarium against lymphedema. Ann Plast Surg 2020;85:e37–43.
2. Schaverien MV, Munnoch DA, Brorson H. Liposuction treatment of lymphedema. Semin Plast Surg 2018;32:42–7.
3. O'Brien BM, Mellow CG, Khazanchi RK, et al. Long-term results after microlymphaticovenous anastomoses for the treatment of obstructive lymphedema. Plast Reconstr Surg 1990;85:562–72.
4. Koshima I, Inagawa K, Urushibara K, et al. Supermicrosurgical lymphaticovenular anastomosis for the treatment of lymphedema in the upper extremities. J Reconstr Microsurg 2000;16:437–42.
5. Schaverien MV, Badash I, Patel KM, et al. Vascularized lymph node transfer for lymphedema. Semin Plast Surg 2018;32:28–35.
6. Johnson AR, Otenti D, Bates KD, et al. Creating a policy for coverage of lymphatic surgery: addressing a critical unmet need. Plast Reconstr Surg 2023. https://doi.org/10.1097/PRS.0000000000010239.
7. The National Lymphoedema Partnership (2019) Commissioning Guidance for Lymphoedema Services for Adults in the United Kingdom. Available at: https://www.thebls.com/documents-library/commissioning-guidance-for-lymphoedema-services-for-adults-in-the-united-kingdom. Accessed 6 March 2023.
8. Markkula SP, Leung N, Allen VB, et al. Surgical interventions for the prevention or treatment of lymphoedema after breast cancer treatment. Cochrane Database Syst Rev 2019;2:CD011433.
9. British Lymphology Society and the Lymphoedema Support Network (2022) Guidelines on the Management of Cellulitis in Lymphoedema. Available at: https://www.thebls.com/documents-library/guidelines-on-the-management-of-cellulitis-in-lymphoedema. Accessed 6 March 2023.
10. Lasinski BB, McKillip Thrift K, Squire D, et al. A systematic review of the evidence for complete decongestive therapy in the treatment of lymphedema from 2004 to 2011. Pharm Manag PM R 2012; 4:580–601.
11. Park KE, Allam O, Chandler L, et al. Surgical management of lymphedema: a review of current literature. Gland Surg 2020;9:503–11.
12. Will PA, Wan Z, Seide SE, et al. Supermicrosurgical treatment for lymphedema: a systematic review and network meta-analysis protocol. Syst Rev 2022;11: 18.
13. Sharkey AR, King SW, Kuo RY, et al. Measuring limb volume: accuracy and reliability of tape measurement versus perometer measurement. Lymphat Res Biol 2018;16:182–6.
14. Basta MN, Gao LL, Wu LC. Operative treatment of peripheral lymphedema: a systematic meta-analysis of the efficacy and safety of lymphovenous microsurgery and tissue transplantation. Plast Reconstr Surg 2014;133:905–13.
15. Carl HM, Walia G, Bello R, et al. Systematic review of the surgical treatment of extremity lymphedema. J Reconstr Microsurg 2017;33:412–25.
16. O'Donnell TF, Allison GM, Iafrati MD. A systematic review of guidelines for lymphedema and the need for contemporary intersocietal guidelines for the management of lymphedema. J Vasc surgery Venous Lymphat Disord 2020;8:676–84.
17. Keeley V, Crooks S, Locke J, et al. A quality of life measure for limb lymphoedema (LYMQOL). J Lymphoedema 2010;5:26–37.
18. Phillips GSA, Gore S, Ramsden A, et al. Lymphaticovenular anastomosis improves quality of life and limb volume in patients with secondary lymphedema after breast cancer treatment. Breast J 2019;25:859–64.
19. Pan WR, Wang DG, Levy SM, et al. Superficial lymphatic drainage of the lower extremity: anatomical study and clinical implications. Plast Reconstr Surg 2013;132:696–707.
20. Chung JH, Baek SO, Park HJ, et al. Efficacy and patient satisfaction regarding lymphovenous bypass with sleeve-in anastomosis for extremity lymphedema. Arch Plast Surg 2019;46:46–56.
21. Narushima M, Koshima I, Mihara M, et al. Intravascular stenting (IVaS) for safe and precise supermicrosurgery. Ann Plast Surg 2008;60:41–4.
22. Ciudad P, Agko M, Perez Coca JJ, et al. Comparison of long-term clinical outcomes among different vascularized lymph node transfers: 6-year experience of a single center's approach to the treatment of lymphedema. J Surg Oncol 2017;116:671–82.
23. Rannikko EH, Suominen SH, Saarikko AM, et al. Long-term results of microvascular lymph node

transfer: correlation of preoperative factors and operation outcome. Plast Reconstr Surg Glob Open 2021;9:e3354.

24. Cha HG, Oh TM, Cho MJ, et al. Changing the paradigm: lymphovenous anastomosis in advanced stage lower extremity lymphedema. Plast Reconstr Surg 2021;147:199–207.

25. Mihara M, Hara H, Kawakami Y, et al. Multi-site lymphatic venous anastomosis using echography to detect suitable subcutaneous vein in severe lymphedema patients. J Plast Reconstr Aesthet Surg 2018;71:e1–7.

26. Seki Y, Kajikawa A, Yamamoto T, et al. Single lymphaticovenular anastomosis for early-stage lower extremity lymphedema treated by the superior-edge-of-the-knee incision method. Plast Reconstr Surg Glob Open 2018;6:e1679.

27. Suzuki Y, Sakuma H, Yamazaki S. Evaluation of patency rates of different lymphaticovenous anastomosis techniques and risk factors for obstruction in secondary upper extremity lymphedema. J Vasc surgery Venous Lymphat Disord 2019;7:113–7.

28. Wolfs JAGN, de Joode LGEH, van der Hulst RRWJ, et al. Correlation between patency and clinical improvement after lymphaticovenous anastomosis (LVA) in breast cancer-related lymphedema: 12-month follow-up. Breast Cancer Res Treat 2020; 179:131–8.

29. Jabbour S, Chang EI. Recent advancements in supermicrosurgical treatment of lymphedema. Plast Aesthet Res 2021;8:43.

30. Mihara M, Hara H, Hayashi Y, et al. Pathological steps of cancer-related lymphedema: histological changes in the collecting lymphatic vessels after lymphadenectomy. PLoS One 2012;7:e41126.

31. Hayashi A, Hayashi N, Yoshimatsu H, et al. Effective and efficient lymphaticovenular anastomosis using preoperative ultrasound detection technique of lymphatic vessels in lower extremity lymphedema. J Surg Oncol 2018;117:290–8.

32. Hayashi A, Yamamoto T, Yoshimatsu H, et al. Ultrasound visualization of the lymphatic vessels in the lower leg. Microsurgery 2016;36:397–401.

33. Hayashi A, Giacalone G, Yamamoto T, et al. Ultra High-frequency ultrasonographic imaging with 70 MHz scanner for visualization of the lymphatic Vessels. Plast Reconstr Surg Glob Open 2019;7:e2086.

34. Bianchi A, Visconti G, Hayashi A, et al. Ultra-High frequency ultrasound imaging of lymphatic channels correlates with their histological features: A step forward in lymphatic surgery. J Plast Reconstr Aesthet Surg 2020;73:1622–9.

35. Boccardo F, Casabona F, De Cian F, et al. Lymphatic microsurgical preventing healing approach (LYMPHA) for primary surgical prevention of breast cancer-related lymphedema: over 4 years follow-up. Microsurgery 2014;34:421–4.

36. DiSipio T, Rye S, Newman B, et al. Incidence of unilateral arm lymphoedema after breast cancer: a systematic review and meta-analysis. Lancet Oncol 2013;14:500–15.

37. Hara Y, Otsubo R, Shinohara S, et al. Lymphedema after axillary lymph node dissection in breast cancer: prevalence and risk factors-a single-center retrospective study. Lymphat Res Biol 2022;20: 600–6.

38. Levy AS, Murphy AI, Ishtihar S, et al. Lymphatic microsurgical preventive healing approach for the primary prevention of lymphedema: a 4-year follow-up. Plast Reconstr Surg 2023;151:413–20.

39. Yang JCS, Wu SC, Lin WC, et al. Supermicrosurgical lymphaticovenous anastomosis as alternative treatment option for moderate-to-severe lower limb lymphedema. J Am Coll Surg 2020;230:216–27.

40. Pandey SK, Fahradyan V, Orfahli LM, et al. Supermicrosurgical lymphaticovenular anastomosis vs. vascularized lymph vessel transplant - technical optimization and when to perform which. Plast Aesthetic Res 2022;8:47.

41. Orfahli LM, Fahradyan V, Chen WF. Vascularized lymph vessel transplant (VLVT): our experience and lymphedema treatment algorithm. Ann Breast Surg 2022;6:8.

42. Head LK, Momtazi M. Economics of lymphovenous bypass. Plast Reconstr Surg 2019;144:751–9.

43. Tom AR, Boudiab E, Issa C, et al. Single center retrospective analysis of cost and payments for lymphatic surgery. Plast Reconstr Surg Glob Open 2021;9:e3630.

44. Dean LT, Moss SL, Ransome Y, et al. "It still affects our economic situation": long-term economic burden of breast cancer and lymphedema. Support Care Cancer 2019;27:1697–708.

Alternative Flap Options for Upper Extremity Reconstruction

Yanis Berkane, MD, MSc[a,b,c,1], Riccardo Giorgino, MD[d,e,f,1], Zhi Yang Ng, MBChB, MRCS, PhD[g], Ruben Dukan, MD, MSc[h], Alexandre G. Lellouch, MD, PhD[b,i,j],*

KEYWORDS

- Upper extremity • Flap reconstruction • DIEP flap • SCIP flap • Microsurgical reconstruction

KEY POINTS

- Various flap techniques exist for the reconstruction of major upper limb defects, with positive outcomes in success rate, function, and esthetics.
- Alternative free flap options exist other than the widely used anterolateral thigh; these include the bipedicled deep inferior epigastric artery perforator flap for extensive defects, and the superficial circumflex iliac artery perforator flap, which represents a newer alternative with promising results.
- Although fasciocutaneous flaps are ideal, their complexity requires case-by-case assessment, and muscle flaps remain a viable alternative.

Video content accompanies this article at http://www.hand.theclinics.com.

INTRODUCTION

The reconstructive approach toward major defects of the upper limb has evolved over time. Muscle flaps have progressively been replaced by fasciocutaneous flaps that show similar or better outcomes with lower morbidity (eg, less tendon adhesions).[1–3] With improvements in surgical techniques and anatomic knowledge, available fasciocutaneous options have evolved even further. They can be used in a variety of configurations, such as free or pedicled and even propeller flaps.[4,5]

When available, pedicled flaps are a reliable solution for defects of the upper extremity.[6] McGregor first described 2-stage pedicled groin flaps[7–9] using neovascularization (or autonomization) principles.[10,11] Although this traditional technique is less commonly used nowadays,[12,13] it

[a] Department of Plastic, Reconstructive and Aesthetic Surgery, CHU Rennes, Rennes University, 16 Boulevard de Bulgarie, 35000 Rennes, France; [b] Vascularized Composite Allotransplantation Laboratory, Massachusetts General Hospital, Harvard Medical School, 50 Blossom Street, Boston, MA 02114, USA; [c] UMR U1236-MICMAC, Immunology and Cell Therapy Lab, Rennes University Hospital, 2 Rue Henri Le Guillou, 35000 Rennes, France; [d] Residency Program in Orthopaedics and Traumatology, University of Milan, Via Cristina Belgioioso, 173, 20161 Milan, Italy; [e] IRCCS Istituto Ortopedico Galeazzi, Via Cristina Belgioioso, 173, 20161 Milan, Italy; [f] Plastic Surgery Research Laboratory, Wellman Center for Photomedicine, Massachusetts General Hospital, Harvard Medical School, 50 Blossom Street, Boston, MA 02114, USA; [g] Department of Plastic and Reconstructive Surgery, John Radcliffe Hospital, Oxford University Hospitals NHS Foundation Trust, Headley Way, Headington, Oxford OX3 9DU, UK; [h] Department of Hand, Upper Limb & Peripheral Nerve Surgery, Georges-Pompidou European Hospital (HEGP), 20 Rue Leblanc, Paris, France; [i] Department of Plastic, Reconstructive & Aesthetic Surgery, Georges-Pompidou European Hospital (HEGP), University of Paris, 20 Rue Leblanc, Paris, France; [j] Innovative Therapies in Haemostasis, INSERM UMR-S 1140, University of Paris, F-75006, Paris, France
[1] Contributed equally.
* Corresponding author. Vascularized Composite Allotransplantation Laboratory, Massachusetts General Hospital, Harvard Medical School, 50 Blossom Street, Boston, MA 02114.
E-mail address: alellouch@mgh.harvard.edu

Hand Clin 40 (2024) 291–299
https://doi.org/10.1016/j.hcl.2023.08.010

has inspired several solutions, such as the superficial inferior epigastric artery,[14] lateral intercostal artery perforator,[15] and paraumbilical flaps.[16] In 1-stage reconstruction, the pedicled thoracodorsal artery perforator (TDAP) flap can be used to cover proximal defects from the axillary fold to the elbow.[17,18] Its pedicle length can be up to 25 cm allowing elbow reconstruction with little to no tension.[19] Other established pedicled options include the lateral arm flap[20,21] and the posterior interosseous artery flap,[22,23] depending on the defect location.

Current free flap options are led by the anterolateral thigh (ALT) flap, which has established itself as the workhorse for the modern reconstruction of major upper limb defects.[24–26] Refinements in recent years have led to improvement of the initial technique with superthin dissection planes,[27] double skin paddles,[28] and turbocharging,[29] thereby improving safety and functional and cosmetic outcomes. This perforator-based approach has been supplemented by similar options, such as the free TDAP[30–32] and, more recently, superficial circumflex iliac artery perforator (SCIP) flaps.[33–35] Finally, the development of the profunda artery perforator (PAP) flap in breast reconstruction has led to alternative, novel use in the upper limb.[36] Further refinements of the PAP flap, with thin and superthin dissection planes, allow the attainment of excellent outcomes and are now used as the procedure of choice in some centers.[37] Such modern perforator flaps require meticulous dissection, and improvements in preoperative planning through computed tomography (CT) angiography and color duplex ultrasonography have emerged.[37,38]

All these microsurgical solutions demand a high level of technical ability and stringent postoperative monitoring protocols but can be limited by the operative time and the patient's overall condition. It is thus critical for the hand surgeon to master several reconstructive techniques. Therefore, the objective of this study is to discuss alternative flap options for major upper limb defect reconstruction through the use of some illustrative case examples.

ALTERNATIVE FLAP OPTIONS

We have selected 4 different flap techniques performed at our centers for patients with major soft tissue defects of the upper limb that required flap surgery (free or pedicled). **Table 1** illustrates the variety of indications and contexts.

Case 1. Free Bipedicled DIEP Flap

The first case describes a 64-year-old woman with type 2 diabetes who suffered a comminuted open

fracture of the left humerus and a degloving injury to her left upper limb in a road traffic accident. The patient was intubated in the emergency department at another institution, where a trauma CT and CT angiography were performed. The CT showed a minor pulmonary embolism but no other injuries were found. The patient was then transferred to our center, where she underwent an exploration of the left brachial artery, followed by thrombectomy and bovine pericardial patch repair performed by the vascular surgeons. An open reduction and internal fixation was then performed on the left radius, with external fixation of the humerus. The external fixation was considered the definitive treatment due to the already compromised soft tissues in a case complicated by coronavirus disease 2019 positivity and underlying diabetes, which increased the risks of infection and delayed healing.

In order to cover the resulting soft tissue defect that was near circumferential (**Fig. 1**A), a free bipedicled deep inferior epigastric artery perforator (DIEP) was performed to resurface the left upper limb. An intraflap anastomosis (end-to-end) was performed between the "opposite" DIEP pedicle to a branch of the main DIEP pedicle, followed by an extraflap anastomosis between the deep inferior epigastric artery (DIEA) and vein (DIEV) to the brachial artery (end-to-side) and the cephalic vein (end-to-end), respectively (**Fig. 1**B). The extended DIEP-based flap allowed for tension-free closure and full coverage of the soft tissue defect (**Fig. 1**C). The donor site was also closed easily as per a standard DIEP procedure (**Fig. 1**D). The patient's postoperative course was otherwise unremarkable, and primary healing was obtained, with a satisfactory esthetic and functional outcome at 1 year of follow-up (**Fig. 1**E). This case illustrates the benefit of the bipedicled technique based on the same principles as supercharging[39-31] and turbocharging,[29,40] improving blood flow through multiple anastomoses to achieve the survival of an extended flap beyond the angiosome of a single perforator. Therefore, the bipedicled DIEP flap can be an option in patients with a moderate-to-high body mass index who have sustained major degloving injuries.[41,42]

Case 2. Pedicled Latissimus Dorsi Flap

Our second patient was a 27-year-old man with ciliary dyskinesia and who was an active smoker. He was the victim of an assault with a firearm (pellet gun) resulting in major trauma of the left arm with extended loss of skin from the mid-arm to the elbow. No significant bone damage was found. Emergent surgical exploration revealed

Table 1
Patient characteristics, flap indications, and outcomes.

Case	Sex	Age (Years)	Comorbidities	Etiology	Flap	Outcome
Patient 1	F	64	T2DM	Comminuted open fracture of the left humerus	Free bipedicled DIEP	Fully healed at 1 y follow-up, able to play piano
Patient 2	M	27	Ciliary dyskinesia, active smoking status	Major trauma of the left arm with extended soft tissue defect from mid-arm to elbow	Pedicled musculocutaneous latissimus dorsi flap	Full healing, physiotherapy after 6 wk, satisfactory functional outcome after 4 mo
Patient 3	M	19	None	Loss of substance after mountain biking accident	Pedicled brachioradialis muscle flap	Full healing after 4 wk (skin graft at wk 3)
Patient 4	F	58	Previous sarcoma of the right forearm, active smoking status	Sarcoma of the right forearm treated with surgery and adjuvant radiotherapy	Free SCIP flap	Full healing after 4 wk

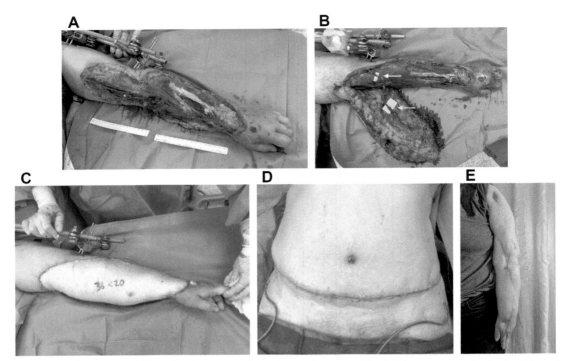

Fig. 1. Case of a 64-year-old female with a comminuted open fracture of the left humerus and degloving injury. A free bipedicled DIEP flap was performed to cover the defect and the material. Consented pictures kindly provided by Mr Marios Nicolaou (Salisbury District Hospital). (*A*) Preoperative presentation with a massive soft tissue defect. The brachial artery and cephalic vein (*white asterisk*) and the extensor digitorum communis tendons (*yellow asterisk*) (*B*) Intraflap anastomosis between the 2 deep inferior epigastric arteries (*yellow arrow*). Anastomosis on the brachial artery (*white arrow*). (*C*) Tension-free closure and full coverage of the soft tissue defect allowed by the extended flap paddle. (*D*) Direct closure of the donor site. (*E*) Final result. Primary healing, with a satisfactory esthetic and functional outcome at 1 year of follow-up.

the absence of the radial pulse, preservation of the ulnar pulse, hypoesthesia of the hand, and subtotal loss of prehension in terms of neurologic signs. Decompression of the radial artery by evacuating a hematoma allowed for flow restoration. No nerve discontinuity was observed in the radial, ulnar, and median nerves. The elbow joint was preserved. After soft tissue debridement, the defect was extensive (**Fig. 2**A).

In view of the potential for partial vascular damage (given the initial loss of radial artery flow), a free flap was considered risky by our team. A pedicled solution was decided on, and because the defect size was major, a musculocutaneous latissimus dorsal (LD) flap was preferred to a TDAP, with the best benefit–risk ratio (short surgery time, safety, and robustness of the flap). The flap was harvested with the patient in an intermediate supine/lateral decubitus position. A vertical skin paddle was drawn to allow for optimal flap inset after 45° of rotation (**Fig. 2**B). The distal tendon of the LD flap was used to reconstruct the distal biceps. Video 1 shows the resulting contraction, eventually allowing restoring flexion of the elbow. A strip of

muscle in the left arm was left exposed to avoid compression of the pedicle (**Fig. 2**C) with the placement of a split-thickness skin graft 2 weeks later. Complete wound healing was achieved, and the patient could start physiotherapy after 6 weeks, with a satisfactory functional outcome at 4 months follow-up (**Fig. 2**D). This case illustrates that while fasciocutaneous free flaps are in vogue for modern upper extremity defect reconstruction, it is still important to consider the robustness of pedicled musculocutaneous flaps.[43] Although a vascularized skin paddle should be preferred for the fold and joint areas to avoid motion range limitation, major defects in the context of emergency can be managed adequately with muscle coverage and delayed skin grafting.[44]

Case 3. Pedicled Brachioradialis Muscle Flap

The third case was that of a 19-year-old man with no past medical history who was involved in a mountain biking accident. He sustained trauma to the right upper limb resulting in an open transolecranon fracture dislocation associated with a

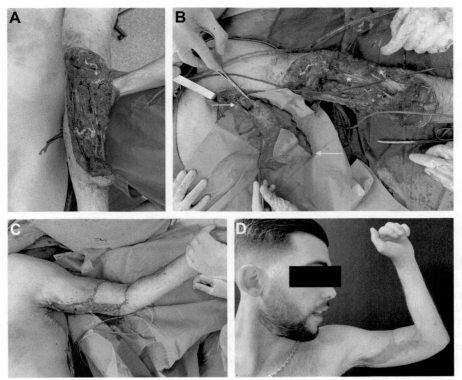

Fig. 2. Case of a 27-year-old man who was the victim of a pellet gun trauma resulting in a major defect of the left arm. A low-risk solution was chosen, and a pedicled musculocutaneous latissimus dorsi (LD) flap was performed. Consented pictures kindly provided by Dr Alexandre G. Lellouch (*A*) Preoperative presentation with an evident soft tissue defect. (*B*) A vertical skin paddle (*yellow arrow*) allowed for optimal flap inset after 45° of rotation with low tension on the pedicle (*white arrow*). No injuries of the vascular axes (brachial artery, *white asterisk*) or nerves were found. The biceps brachii was partially preserved (*yellow asterisk*). (*C*) A strip of the LD muscle was left exposed (*black asterisk*) in the medial arm to avoid compression of the pedicle. (*D*) Final result. Complete wound healing, with a satisfactory esthetic and functional outcome at 4 months follow-up.

closed comminuted distal radius fracture. His initial surgery was performed at a local facility where he had sustained the injury, using an external fixator. The patient then presented to our center at postoperative day 15 with a wound infection and was taken to the OR. After debridement, an open reduction and osteosynthesis of the olecranon was performed using a screwed plate (Variax, Stryker, Michigan, USA; **Fig. 3**A). A brachioradialis muscle flap (**Fig. 3**B) associated with a local rotation skin flap was then used for hardware coverage. Additional acellular dermal matrix (ADM; Duragen, Integra Lifescience, Princeton, NJ) was applied and affixed with staples (**Fig. 3**C). The distal radial fracture was reduced and fixed with a volar locking plate (Aptus, Medartis, Bale, Switzerland). The joint surface was reduced under arthroscopic control and fixed with K-wires. A split-thickness skin graft was performed 3 weeks after application of the ADM, and full wound healing was obtained after

4 weeks. No complication was reported, and the patient achieved a satisfactory range of motion (flexion 130°, extension −20°, pronation 80°, and supination 80°; **Fig. 3**D). This case emphasizes the usefulness of local muscle flaps that represent an efficient solution in such difficult situations by obtaining well-vascularized tissue for coverage and providing an optimal wound bed for skin grafting.[43] The brachioradialis flap has been described as an alternative for posterior elbow wounds.[45] In addition, to improve the quality of the healed tissue, ADM has proven to be a valuable tool in the upper extremity.[46,47]

Case 4. Free Superficial Circumflex Iliac Artery Perforator Flap

Finally, the last patient was a 58-year-old woman who was treated 4 months previously for a right forearm sarcoma with surgery and postoperative adjuvant radiotherapy who then presented with

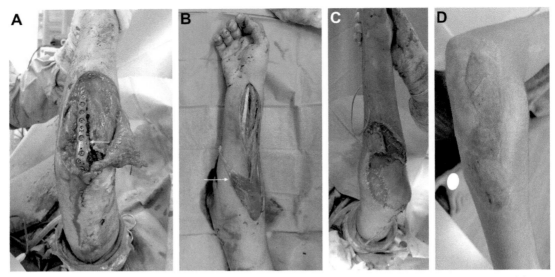

Fig. 3. Case of a 19-year-old man with an open trans-olecranon fracture initially treated with an external fixator. A wound infection led to debridement, screwed-plate-based osteosynthesis, and the resulting defect was covered by a combination of a pedicled brachioradialis flap and an ADM before skin grafting. (*A*) Open reduction and osteosynthesis of the olecranon with a screwed plate (Variax, Stryker, Michigan, USA) (*yellow arrow*) performed after debridement. (*B*) Brachioradialis muscle flap (*white arrow*) associated with a local rotation skin flap. (*C*) ADM (Duragen, Integra Lifescience, Princeton, NJ) was applied to enhance healing and was affixed with staples. (*D*) Final result. Full healing, with a satisfactory esthetic and functional outcome at 4 weeks follow-up.

radiodermatitis and consequent exposure of the underlying radius (**Fig. 4**A). Unfortunately, the patient was still actively smoking. After a multidisciplinary team discussion, wide soft tissue resection with bone trimming was decided upon, followed by 1-stage soft tissue coverage. Given the location of the defect, a free SCIP flap raised along the superficial fat layer above the superficial fascia, in erthin

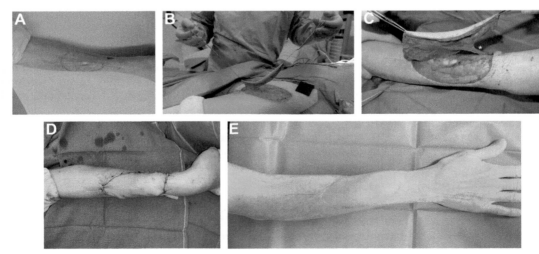

Fig. 4. Case of a 58-year-old woman presenting with radiodermatitis and bone exposure following radiotherapy. A wide soft tissue resection with bone trimming was performed, and the defect was covered using a free thin SCIP flap, resulting in optimal coverage. Consented pictures kindly provided by Dr. Paul Girard and Pr. Nicolas Bertheuil (CHU de Rennes). (*A*) Radiodermatitis and exposure of the radius after surgery and postoperative adjuvant radiotherapy. (*B*) Free SCIP flap raised in the thin plane. (*C*) Harvesting of the flap on the superficial branch of the superficial circumflex iliac artery (SCIA, *white asterisk*). (*D*) Final positioning of the flap with the vessels (SCIA) anastomosed end-to-side to the radial artery and accompanying venae comitantes. (*E*) Final result. Full healing, with an excellent esthetic outcome at 4 weeks of follow-up.

fashion, was chosen (**Fig. 4**B). The flap was harvested on the superficial branch of the SCIA only, and the vessels were anastomosed end-to-side to the radial artery and accompanying venae comitantes (**Fig. 4**C, D). No postoperative complication occurred, and the patient's wound had fully healed after 4 weeks. The result was found to be excellent, with minimal contour deformity of the flap in the forearm after 1 year (**Fig. 4**E). The flap's thinness also allowed the patient to resume her usual activities. The donor site healed without complication. The SCIP flap shows high adaptability through the variable thickness, adjustable pedicle length, and flap dimensions.[33,34]

DISCUSSION

These selected cases demonstrate the effectiveness of various modern reconstructive techniques for major defects of the upper limbs resulting from various causes, with high technical success, satisfactory functional and esthetic results, and a low rate of complications. Therefore, the modern hand and reconstructive microsurgeon should keep in mind that alternative solutions, both pedicled and free, do exist besides well-established approaches such as the ALT and TDAP flaps.

LIMITATIONS

One critical parameter missing in our case series and poorly described in the literature is assessing the quality of life following upper limb reconstruction. It could be highly informative to assess function and quality of life using validated questionnaires, such as the upper extremity function test or the Sollerman hand function test, to better objectively assess the outcomes of all different alternatives. That, however, is beyond the scope of the current article.

SUMMARY

In conclusion, the discussion around this series of patient cases demonstrates the efficacy of various flap reconstruction techniques for major upper limb defects, with favorable outcomes regarding success rate and functional and esthetic results. Bipedicled DIEP flaps can be used for selected patients with extensive defects. Various refinements can improve ALT flaps to reach even better outcomes, whereas SCIP flaps represent an attractive newer alternative providing high-quality results. Reconstructive surgeons have a range of solutions at their disposal, among which fasciocutaneous flaps are generally considered the most optimal given the functional requirements of the hand. However, technical sophistication and complexity of these options require a case-by-case assessment. Simpler solutions, such as pedicled musculocutaneous flaps combined with skin grafts, should also be part of our armamentarium to ensure that patient outcomes are not compromised regardless of the circumstances.

CLINICS CARE POINTS

- Alternative flap options for the reconstruction of major defects of the upper limb can be used successfully.
- Bipedicled DIEP flaps can be an adequate solution for extensive and deep defects in patients with soft tissue excess at the donor site.
- Pedicled myocutaneous/muscle flaps such as the latissimus dorsi and brachioradialis flaps are invaluable options in cases where microsurgery may not be suitable.
- Newer techniques, such as free SCIP flaps, are challenging but can provide superior results in selected patients.

ACKNOWLEDGMENTS

The authors would like to acknowledge Marios Nicolaou from the Odstock Regional Center for Burns, Plastic and Reconstructive Surgery, Salisbury District Hospital, Wiltshire, United Kingdom, for providing consented pictures of the patient discussed in case 1, and Pr Nicolas Bertheuil and Dr Paul Girard from Rennes University Hospital Center, France for providing consented pictures of the patient discussed in case 4.

DISCLOSURE

The authors have nothing to disclose.

SUPPLEMENTARY DATA

Supplementary data related to this article can be found online at https://doi.org/10.1016/j.hcl.2023.08.010.

REFERENCES

1. Ng ZY, Tan SSY, Lellouch AG, et al. Soft Tissue Reconstruction of Complete Circumferential Defects of the Upper Extremity. Archives of plastic surgery 2017;44(2):117–23.
2. Ng ZY, Salgado CJ, Moran SL, et al. Soft tissue coverage of the mangled upper extremity. Semin Plast Surg 2015;29(1):48–54.

3. Ng ZY, Askari M, Chim H. Approach to complex upper extremity injury: an algorithm. Semin Plast Surg 2015;29(1):5–9.

4. Kovar A, Colakoglu S, Iorio ML. A Systematic Review of Muscle and Fasciocutaneous Flaps in the Treatment of Extremity Osteomyelitis: Evidence for Fasciocutaneous Flap Use. Plastic and Reconstructive Surgery – Global Open 2019;7:1–2.

5. Vitse J, Bekara F, Bertheuil N, et al. Perforator-based propeller flaps reliability in upper extremity soft tissue reconstruction: a systematic review. J Hand Surg Eur 2017;42:157–64.

6. Sananpanich K, Tu YK, Kraisarin J, et al. Reconstruction of limb soft-tissue defects: using pedicle perforator flaps with preservation of major vessels, a report of 45 cases. Injury 2008;39(Suppl 4):55–66.

7. McGregor IA. Basic principles in skin flap transfer. Surg Clin North Am 1977;57:961–76.

8. McGregor IA. Flap reconstruction in hand surgery: the evolution of presently used methods. J Hand Surg Am 1979;4:1–10.

9. McGregor IA, Jackson IT. The groin flap. Br J Plast Surg 1972;25:3–16.

10. Giordano L, Galli A, Familiari M, et al. Head and neck pedicled flap autonomization using a new high-resolution indocyanine green fluorescence video-angiography device. Head Neck 2022;44(6):1496–9.

11. Berkane Y, Alana Shamlou A, Reyes J, et al. The Superficial Inferior Epigastric Artery Axial Flap to Study Ischemic Preconditioning Effects in a Rat Model. J Vis Exp 2023;191.

12. Rubio-Gallegos F, Núñez-González S, Gault C, et al. McGregor inguinal flap for coverage of large soft tissue losses due to high-voltage electrical burns in the upper limb: a retrospective study. Int J Burns Trauma 2019;9:52–8.

13. Buchman SJ, Eglseder WA Jr, Robertson BC. Pedicled groin flaps for upper-extremity reconstruction in the elderly: a report of 4 cases. Arch Phys Med Rehabil 2002;83:850–4.

14. Habib ME, Reuter CH. Bilateral Pedicled Superficial Epigastric Flap in the Management of Circumferential Combined Degloving and Full Thickness Burn Hand Injury™A Case Report. Mod Plast Surg 2012;02:4.

15. Yunchuan P, Jiaqin X, Sihuan C, et al. Use of the Lateral Intercostal Perforator-Based Pedicled Abdominal Flap for Upper-Limb Wounds From Severe Electrical Injury. Ann Plast Surg 2006;56:116–21.

16. Kamath BJ, Verghese T, Bhardwaj P. "Wing flaps": perforator-based pedicled paraumbilical flaps for skin defects in hand and forearm. Ann Plast Surg 2007;59:495–500.

17. Ete G, Paul K, Akamanchi AK, et al. Pedicled thoracodorsal artery perforator flap in the soft-tissue reconstruction of an acute traumatic cubital fossa defect. J Plast Reconstr Aesthet Surg 2022;75:2070–6.

18. Oksüz S, Ulkür E, Tuncer S, et al. Elbow reconstruction with a pedicled thoracodorsal artery perforator flap after excision of an upper-extremity giant hairy nevus. J Plast Reconstr Aesthet Surg 2013;66:566–9.

19. Kulahci Y, Sahin C, Karagoz H, et al. Pre-expanded Thoracodorsal Artery Perforator Flap. Clin Plast Surg 2017;44:91–7.

20. Heidekrueger PI, Mueller C, Thiha A, et al. The lateral arm flap for reconstruction of tissue defects due to olecranon bursitis. J Plast Surg Hand Surg 2018;52:347–51.

21. Innocenti M, Baldrighi C, Delcroix L, et al. Local perforator flaps in soft tissue reconstruction of the upper limb. Handchir Mikrochir Plast Chir 2009;41:315–21.

22. Engelbrecht JJ, Bruce-Chwatt AJ. The posterior interosseous flap for soft-tissue cover of the hand. S Afr J Surg 1996;34:194–6.

23. Zaidenberg EE, Zancolli P, Farias Cisneros E, et al. Antegrade Posterior Interosseous Flap for Nonhealing Wounds of the Elbow: Anatomical and Clinical Study. Plastic and Reconstructive Surgery – Global Open 2018;6:e1959.

24. Gupta A, Lakhiani C, Lim BH, et al. Free tissue transfer to the traumatized upper extremity: Risk factors for postoperative complications in 282 cases. J Plast Reconstr Aesthet Surg 2015;68:1184–90.

25. Koteswara Rao Rayidi V, Prakash P, Srikanth R, et al. Anterolateral Thigh Flap-the Optimal Flap in Coverage of Severe Elbow Injuries. Indian J Plast Surg 2019;52:314–21.

26. Yang Z, Xu C, Zhu Y, et al. Flow-Through Free Anterolateral Thigh Flap in Reconstruction of Severe Limb Injury. Ann Plast Surg 2020;84:S165–70.

27. Cha HG, Hur J, Ahn C, et al. Ultra-Thin Anterolateral Thigh Free Flap: An Adipocutaneous Flap with the Most Superficial Elevation Plane. Plast Reconstr Surg 2023.

28. He J, Qing L, Wu P, et al. Customized reconstruction of complex soft tissue defects in the upper extremities with variants of double skin paddle anterolateral thigh perforator flap. Injury 2021;52:1771–7.

29. Lee YJ, Lee YJ, Oh DY, et al. Reconstruction of wide soft tissue defects with extended anterolateral thigh perforator flap turbocharged technique with anteromedial thigh perforator. Microsurgery 2020;40:440–6.

30. Chang LS, Kim YH, Kim SW. Reconstruction of burn scar contracture deformity of the extremities using thin thoracodorsal artery perforator free flaps. ANZ J Surg 2021;91:E578–83.

31. Lee SH, Mun GH. Transverse thoracodorsal artery perforator flaps: experience with 31 free flaps. J Plast Reconstr Aesthet Surg 2008;61:372–9.

32. Miyamoto S, Arikawa M, Kagaya Y, et al. Septocutaneous thoracodorsal artery perforator flaps: a retrospective cohort study. J Plast Reconstr Aesthet Surg 2019;72:78–84.

33. Berner JE, Nikkhah D, Zhao J, et al. The Versatility of the Superficial Circumflex Iliac Artery Perforator Flap: A Single Surgeon's 16-Year Experience for Limb Reconstruction and a Systematic Review. J Reconstr Microsurg 2020;36:93–103.

34. S A, D B. Multifarious uses of the pedicled SCIP flap - a case series. Acta Chir Plast 2023;64:148–54.

35. Visconti G, Bianchi A, Salgarello M. The use of the distal posterior radial collateral artery as recipient vessel in elbow resurfacing using SCIP flap. Microsurgery 2021;41:699–700.

36. Boriani F, Sassu P, Atzeni M, et al. The profunda artery perforator flap for upper limb reconstruction: A case report and literature review on the flap applications in reconstruction. Microsurgery 2022;42:714–21.

37. Chim H. Perforator mapping and clinical experience with the superthin profunda artery perforator flap for reconstruction in the upper and lower extremities. J Plast Reconstr Aesthet Surg 2023;81:60–7.

38. Yoshimatsu H, Karakawa R, Fuse Y, et al. Superficial Circumflex Iliac Artery Perforator Flap Elevation Using Preoperative High-Resolution Ultrasonography for Vessel Mapping and Flap Design. J Reconstr Microsurgery 2022;38(3):217–20.

39. Agarwal P, Sharma D, Kukrele R. Arteriovenous supercharging: A novel approach to improve reliability of the distally based sural flap. Trop Doct 2021;51:339–44.

40. Semple JL. Retrograde microvascular augmentation (turbocharging) of a single-pedicle TRAM flap through a deep inferior epigastric arterial and venous loop. Plast Reconstr Surg 1994;93:109–17.

41. Zhang W, Zhu W, Li X, et al. Effects of Distal Arterial Supercharging and Distal Venous Superdrainage on the Survival of Multiterritory Perforator Flaps in Rats. J Invest Surg 2022;35:1462–71.

42. Ou Q, Wu P, Zhou Z, et al. Algorithm for covering circumferential wound on limbs with ALTP or/and DIEP flaps based on chain-linked design and combined transplantation. Injury 2021;52:1356–62.

43. Hihara M, Kuro A, Mitsui T, et al. Twenty-minute harvesting of flow-through type vastus lateralis muscle flap significantly reduces the need for a temporary intravascular shunt in the treatment of severe upper extremity trauma in civilian patients. Medicine (Baltim) 2023;102:e33311.

44. He J, Qing L, Wu P, et al. Variations of Extended Latissimus Dorsi Musculocutaneous Flap for Reconstruction of Large Wounds in the Extremity. Orthop Surg 2022;14:2598–606.

45. Sabbag OD, DeDeugd CM, Wagner ER, et al. Brachioradialis Flap for Soft Tissue Coverage of Posterior Elbow Wounds: Case Report and Surgical Technique. Tech Hand Up Extrem Surg 2019;1:2–5.

46. Fonzone Caccese F, Crisci E, Lanzano G, et al. Reconstruction of the degloved dorsal wrist using a combination of a local adipofascial flap and acellular dermal matrix. J Hand Surg Eur 2023;48:361–3.

47. Ali B, Wu J, Borah G, et al. Temporary Use of Acellular Dermal Matrix in Upper Extremity Salvage. Plast Reconstr Surg Glob Open 2020;8(7):e2965.

Simultaneous or Delayed Free Tissue Transfer in Combination with Replantation Surgery

Soo Jin Woo, MD, Kwang Hyun Park, MD, Sang Hyun Woo, MD, PhD*

KEYWORDS

• Replantation • Simultaneous free flap • Delayed free flap • Reconstruction

KEY POINTS

- The primary objectives of simultaneous free flap reconstruction during replantation are to ensure the survival of the amputated digit or hand and to provide tissue for faster wound healing by restoring anatomic structures. In digit replantation, the arterialized venous flap proves indispensable by offering vessel conduits and soft tissue coverage together.
- In cases of major limb amputations where bone shortening is performed during replantation, the requirement for vessel conduits often becomes redundant. Here, a simultaneous free flap provides soft tissue to cover exposed essential structures like tendons, bones, and joints.
- In delayed reconstruction, the main objective is the enhancement of function. Consideration may be given to free flaps that incorporate bone, joint, and nerve components in addition to soft tissue. A free functioning muscle transfer is the most powerful tool for restoring flexion and extension in the hand and upper extremity. For large bone defects, a vascularized fibular flap can play a crucial role in augmenting function.

INTRODUCTION

Traumatic amputations of the hand and upper extremity can profoundly affect a patient's quality of life, as they bear significant psychological and physical sequelae. Maintaining functional capacity often necessitates intricate reconstruction of digits, hand, forearm, and upper arm, which entail not only replantation but also free flap procedures. This article explores the various free flaps used during and after replantation, with the aim of enhancing understanding of replantation results and aiding the surgical decision-making processes.

Published literature regarding the timing for extremity reconstruction after trauma continues to show significant variation, with investigators suggesting different timelines[1–6] (**Table 1**). In this article, the authors have organized the content into two sections. Simultaneous reconstruction refers to procedures that are performed concurrently or shortly after replantation while the wound from the injury is still present. Delayed reconstruction refers to procedures that are performed after replantation and other initial surgeries, once the wound from the initial injury has completely closed.

The aim of using a free flap for simultaneous reconstruction with replantation is to restore the physiologic circulation of the amputated site to ensure survival, or to achieve wound healing through anatomic restoration. Delayed reconstruction using a free flap is intended to enhance the functional improvement or cosmetic acceptance of a replanted part.

W Institute for Hand and Reconstructive Microsurgery, W General Hospital, Daegu, South Korea
* Corresponding author. 1632 Dalgubeol-daero, Dalseo-gu, Daegu 42642, South Korea.
E-mail address: handwoo303@gmail.com

Hand Clin 40 (2024) 301–313
https://doi.org/10.1016/j.hcl.2023.08.013

Table 1
Nomenclature for free flap based on timing and purpose of reconstruction

Author, Year of Publication	Definition
Based on the Time of Event (Injury or Replantation)	
Godina,[6] 1986	Early reconstruction: Free flap transfer within 72 h of injury Delay reconstruction: Free flap transfer between 72 h and 3 mo after injury Late reconstruction: Free flap transfer performed more than 3 mo after injury
Lister & Schecker,[1] 1988	Emergency free flap: Procedures performed at the end of the primary debridement, within 24 h of the time of the injury
Derderian et al,[2] 2003	Emergency free tissue transfer: Procedures performed emergently at the time of injury Early primary free tissue transfer: Procedures performed either emergently at the time of injury, during 1–5 d after injury Delayed primary tissue transfer: Procedures performed during 6–21 d after injury Late free tissue transfer: Procedures performed 21 d after injury
Ninkovic et al,[3] 1999	Primary free flap closure: Closure with free flap at the end of initial radical debridement or within 24 h Delayed primary free flap closure: Closure with free flap at 2–7 d after creation of defect Secondary free flap closure: Closure with free flap beyond 1 wk
Yu et al,[4] 2003 (classification on secondary procedures in replantation surgery)	Early procedures: Procedures within 2 mo following replantation Late procedures: Procedures after 2 mo following replantation
Based on the Purpose of Surgical Procedure	
Sabapathy & Bhardwaj,[5] 2013 (classification on secondary procedures in replantation surgery)	Group 1: Procedures to restore continuity of structures that were not repaired during the primary procedure Group 2: Procedures to promote healing or enhance function of structures repaired during the original procedure Group 3: Procedures not part of the normal steps of replantation but which are done secondarily to enhance function and cosmesis

SIMULTANEOUS RECONSTRUCTION USING FREE FLAP WITH REPLANTATION

Following Godina's pioneering work in the 1980s,[6] which conceptualized the use of "emergency" free flaps, free tissue transfer has been used not only for closing acute wounds but also for complete reconstruction after the initial injury. Although the focus remains on maximizing tissue preservation and replantation where feasible, a multitude of concurrent concerns must also be addressed. Simultaneous reconstruction through a free flap

with replantation offers a potent strategy not just addressing the loss of soft tissue but also assuring the survival of the replanted part.

Indications

Simultaneous free flap reconstruction is primarily indicated in two situations. First, a free flap can provide a vessel conduit for cases with a vessel defect in incomplete or complete amputations.[7,8] When ruptured arteries cannot be approximated owing to excessive tension or a segmental gap, alternative strategies, such as interposition vein grafts or use of an undamaged adjacent artery, are considered. Free flaps can also be used as flow-through vascular conduits, enabling both soft tissue coverage and vascular reconstruction. A composite free flap can offer the advantage of incorporating tissues, including vessels, bone, joint, tendon, or nerves. However, apart from the vascular defect, tissues such as bone, joint, tendon, and nerve are not usually reconstructed in a simultaneous setting. Instead, bone deficits are managed with bone cement, tendons are addressed with artificial tendons using silicone rods, and nerves are initially tagged for subsequent nerve grafting.

Second, a free flap can provide vascularized coverage for wounds that involve the exposure of vessels, nerves, joints, tendons without paratenon, or bone without periosteum. Other options, such as vacuum-assisted closure for negative pressure wound therapy or skin grafts, can cause excessive granulation and scar formation over tendons and adhesion to the underlying structure, which leads to limitation of motion.[9] On the other hand, local, regional, and distant flaps can provide soft tissue coverage. However, they have inherent limitations in size and reach and may prolong immobilization.[10]

Contraindications for simultaneous reconstruction include cases where stable skeletal support cannot be achieved in a single stage or patients who are medically unstable and unable to tolerate an extended surgical procedure.

Advantages and Essentials of Simultaneous Free Flap Reconstruction

The benefits of simultaneous free flap reconstruction extend beyond addressing vessel defects and providing immediate coverage to essential structures. It reduces the number of surgical procedures, allows for shorter hospital stays offering psychological benefits to the patients, and facilitates early initiation of rehabilitation and mobilization.[11,12] Although earlier studies suggested that performing microsurgical reconstruction within 24 to 72 hours of injury can lower the infection rate and flap failure,[1,6,13] recent studies have shown that timing of free flap reconstruction does not significantly impact both outcomes.[14]

Technical advantages are evident during simultaneous free flap reconstruction, particularly when performed immediately after the injury. At this early stage, dissection of tissue planes is easier due to minimal fibrosis and edema. The injured vessels near the wound still maintain robust blood flow, making them suitable for use as recipient vessels. Delayed reconstruction presents challenges, such as prolonged artery spasm and increased risk of tearing and narrowing in venae comitantes.

Before attempting simultaneous free flap reconstruction, radical debridement of all nonviable and necrotic tissue is essential.[6] This step transforms a contaminated wound into a clean one, mitigating the risk of infection and providing an opportunity to assess the extent of injury and predict reconstructive requirements. If radical debridement is not feasible, simultaneous free flap reconstruction is unsafe as the definitive reconstruction and should be performed when the wound is free from infection. The risk of serious infection is a crucial consideration because it threatens the free flap, the limb, and finally, the quality of functional recovery.

Another principle is ensuring a safe vascular anastomosis. Ideally, the anastomosis should be done proximal to the zone of injury. However, certain studies have reported favorable outcomes with distal or even in-zone anastomosis for soft tissue reconstruction of digits.[15,16] Anastomosis should be done after adequate resection of the proximal vessel and assessment of blood spurting from the cut end. Continuous spasm or weak spurting indicates damage to the proximal artery, necessitating further resection until a pulsatile flow is observed.[17] In most cases, the arterial anastomosis is performed before venous repair to minimize ischemic time. This approach facilitates the filling of dorsal veins, assisting in the identification of delicate veins and other recipient vessels for simultaneous reconstruction. During simultaneous free flap reconstruction, it is important to avoid impeding vascularization of the replanted tissue. Harvesting a flap with a long pedicle can facilitate anastomosis at a distant location, potentially necessitating the use of vein grafts or end-to-side anastomosis.

Free Flap Options for Simultaneous Reconstruction with Replantation

Various free flap options for simultaneous reconstruction are listed and discussed based on clinical cases, categorized by the level of amputation: digit, hand/wrist, forearm/upper arm.

Digital defect
Restoration of digital artery using an arterialized venous flap A flow-through flap with a vessel conduit can deliver the dual benefits of vascular reconstruction and soft tissue coverage. Among various flaps with a flow-through conduit, venous flaps are advantageous for use in the digits owing to several characteristics (**Fig. 1**).[7,8,18] A venous flap can be harvested from the volar aspect of the forearm or distal wrist, including the thenar

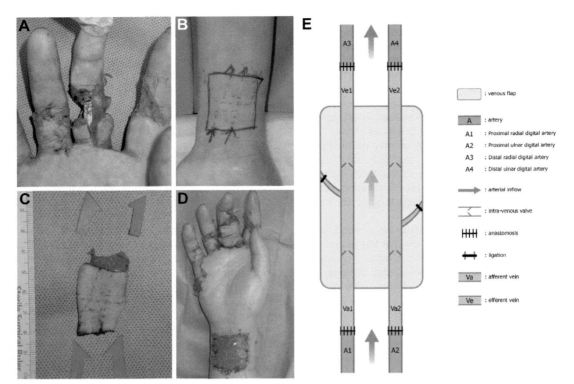

Fig. 1. This 30-year-old man sustained multiple punch-out injuries on his right hand from a press machine. (*A*) The right middle finger was incompletely amputated with flexor tendon rupture in zone 2 and a soft tissue defect with 2.5-cm and 3-cm missing segments at the ulnar digital artery and radial digital artery, respectively. Debridement was followed by a flexor digitorum profundus tendon tenorrhaphy and temporary immobilization of the PIP joint using a single K-wire preceding the free flap inset. (*B*) A 3.5 × 5-cm sized venous flap with 4 veins was harvested from the ipsilateral wrist. (*C*) The flap was designed with two sets of through-valve types, establishing a flow-through venous pattern. The afferent veins were repaired to the proximal ulnar and radial digital arteries, whereas the efferent veins were repaired to their respective distal ulnar and radial digital arteries. Two efferent veins were anastomosed to two subcutaneous veins in the digit for venous drainage. (*D*) The donor site was covered with a split-thickness skin graft from the plantar aspect of the foot. Both the flap and the replanted finger distal to the flap survived without any complications. (*E*) Schematic diagram describes the vessel anastomosis. *Courtesy* of Myung-Jae Yoo.

area in one operating field under one tourniquet. It provides thin and pliable coverage of the digit with good contour without the need for secondary debulking procedures.[8,19] An arterialized venous flap can also take different forms, such as a tendo-cutaneous venous flap using palmaris longus tendon, innervated venous flap using cutaneous nerve, or composite flap to manage compound tissue defects.[8,20,21]

Coverage of the palmar side of the digit using a radial artery superficial palmar branch flap A simultaneous free flap can be used not only to address the vessel deficit but also to provide immediate coverage. Soft tissue defects can occur owing to the injury itself, by radical debridement performed alongside replantation, or by partial loss of replanted tissue after a successful replantation. In traction avulsion injuries and crushing

injuries, distally and proximally based skin flaps have low survival rates[22] owing to damaged microcirculation and their distance from the neo-vascularized blood supply (**Fig. 2**). It is not uncommon to observe partial tissue necrosis starting 7 days after the initial operation, leading to exposure of vital structures, such as an artery, vein graft, or repaired nerve. Also, the long-term viability of revascularized digital arteries varies with approximately 37% of vessels experiencing artery occlusion within an average of 15 days postoperatively.[23] A free flap can facilitate prompt and effective soft tissue healing, which is crucial for the development of new blood vessels in the replanted tissue. Particularly in crush injuries, the process of neovascularization in the replanted tissue tends to be slow, thereby increasing the risk of partial tissue necrosis occurring between 7 and 10 days after the operation.[17]

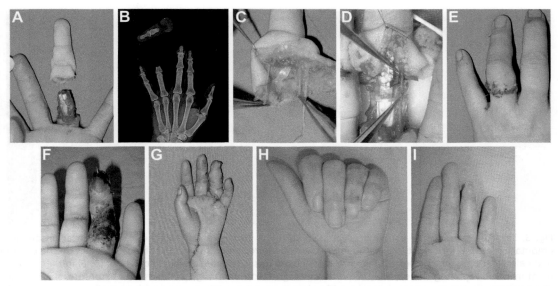

Fig. 2. A 43-year-old woman presented with a left ring finger avulsion amputation caused by a wire mesh of a hen house. (*A*, *B*) The left ring finger was completely avulsed at the proximal third of the middle phalangeal bone with an intact PIP joint. (*C*) Both the radial and the ulnar digital arteries showed ribbon signs, and the digital nerves were avulsed. (*D*) Following the reduction and fixation of the middle phalanx, flexor digitorum profundus tendon tenorrhaphy was done. The ulnar digital artery was repaired using a 1.2-cm vein graft at the volar aspect of the PIP joint, and one dorsal vein was repaired. Because of the defect in both digital nerves, the proximal radial digital nerve was transposed to the distal ulnar digital nerve. (*E*) Immediate postoperative photograph. (*F*) Four weeks after the initial operation, there was partial loss of soft tissue around the volar side of the PIP joint area and the pulp of the finger. (*G*) After debridement of the necrotic tissue, a 3 × 7-cm radial artery superficial palmar branch flap was harvested from the ipsilateral thenar area to resurface the palmar side of the ring finger. Artery anastomosis was performed end to end with the common palmar digital artery between the third and fourth metacarpal, and the vein was repaired to a subcutaneous vein. The donor site was closed primarily. (*H*, *I*) Twenty months after the operation. *Courtesy of Ho-Jun Cheon.*

The palmar side of the digits has a sturdy nature, making glabrous flaps, such as the radial artery superficial palmar branch flap,[24] toe pulp flap,[25] thenar flap,[26] and hypothenar flap,[27] potential options. Other durable flaps, such as the anterolateral thigh flap, medial pedis flap, and lateral arm flap, may be too thick and bulky to resurface this area. If feasible, a sensate flap can further improve outcomes and enhance patient satisfaction. If a similar sized defect to this case is on the dorsum of the finger, it is preferable to consider flaps that are thin and elastic to facilitate joint motion, such as an arterialized venous flap, dorsalis pedis flap,[28] superficial circumflex iliac artery perforator flap,[29] and first web space of foot flap.[30]

Hand and wrist defect
Coverage of both palmar and dorsal sides of the wrist joint using a split anterolateral thigh flap
Replantation at the level of the radiocarpal joint usually involves bone shortening depending on the involved joint and the level of amputation, which can allow for direct repair of vessels, nerves, and primary soft tissue closure. For amputations at the intercarpal or radiocarpal joint level with an intact distal articular surface, proximal row carpectomy is done leading to an overall shortening effect of 2 to 3 cm. In situations with extensive bone fractures around the radiocarpal joint, partial or total carpectomy and primary arthrodesis of the wrist are performed.[31] When the amputation is just above the distal articular surface of the radius, a radial shortening osteotomy and a Darrach procedure are performed.[31] If soft tissue defects remain even after bone shortening, a simultaneous free flap can be used to cover the exposed bone, joint, or hardware.

When the defect involves both the palmar and the dorsal sides of the hand, such as in the case shown in **Fig. 3**, or when irregularly shaped defects are present, a wider flap can be harvested and then trimmed to fit the defect, or two separate flaps can be used. However, these approaches may increase donor-site morbidity and hinder achieving primary closure leading to lower patient satisfaction.[32] Splitting the flap based on different

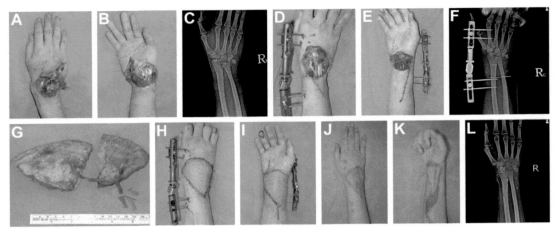

Fig. 3. This 20-year-old man experienced a crushing injury from a press machine, resulting in an incomplete amputation at the right wrist. (*A, B*) The injury created a through-and-through soft tissue defect on the dorsum and palm. (*C*) The plain radiograph revealed carpal bone loss with radiocarpal dissociation. (*D, E*) Initial management involved repairing the ulnar artery with a vein graft, common digital nerves, and extensor pollicis longus and extensor digitorum communis tendons. The defect was temporarily covered with an acellular dermal matrix. (*F*) Postoperative radiograph showed reduction and fixation of the distal radius metaphysis with K-wires, and the radiocarpal joint was stabilized with an additional external fixator. (*G*) The following day, simultaneous reconstruction was performed using a single anterolateral thigh flap with two different perforators from the same pedicle perfusing different skin paddles. (*H, I*) The flap was split and reshaped to cover the dorsal and palmar defects. Microanastomosis was performed to the radial artery, and venous anastomosis was completed to a superficial vein. The flap survived without any complications. (*J–L*) Postoperative photographs and radiograph after 6 months. *Courtesy* of Dong-Ho Kang.

sizable perforators allows for precise tailoring and coverage of irregularly shaped defects with only one pedicle, while still being able to close the donor site primarily (see **Fig. 3**).[33] Flaps such as the anterolateral flap, radial forearm flap, and lateral arm flap have distinct cutaneous perforators with independent territories and can be split for use.[34]

Forearm and upper arm defect

Simultaneous reconstruction of the ulnar using a fibular flap and delayed reconstruction of finger flexion using a free functioning gracilis muscle transfer A major limb amputation is defined as an amputation that occurs at or proximal to the radiocarpal joint, encompassing transections at levels including the wrist, forearm, elbow, humerus, or shoulder. Because of the critical constraint of keeping total ischemia time within 8 hours, the initial operation should prioritize successful revascularization over introducing additional complexity with free flap procedures. Coverage of the anastomosed vessel with a skin flap must be ensured, whereas the other tissues can be temporarily protected using an artificial dermis or a skin graft.

After securing the survival of replanted tissue and depending on the patients' general condition, the necessary free flap reconstruction is performed within the first week. For defects involving the radius or ulna bones, vascularized bone flap, such as fibular flap, can be considered (**Fig. 4**). The fibular flap is widely favored owing to its ease of access, reliable pedicle, and ability to provide a significant length of bone without compromising leg function, as well as its ability to provide a reliable skin paddle.[35] For soft tissue defects, perforator flaps, such as the posterior interosseous artery perforator flap, superficial circumflex iliac artery perforator flap, and lateral arm perforator flap, are suitable for providing extensive and thin coverage.[36] Although cutaneous flaps are often used for upper extremity coverage, some prefer myocutaneous flaps for filling dead space, making them suitable for large and deep wounds. Conversely, muscle flaps, such as the latissimus dorsi flap, rectus abdominis muscle flap, and serratus anterior muscle flap, with split-thickness skin grafts are not recommended owing to difficulties in flap reelevation and closure during secondary surgical procedures.

DELAYED RECONSTRUCTION USING FREE FLAP AFTER REPLANTATION

Delayed reconstruction takes place once the wound from the initial injury has been covered.

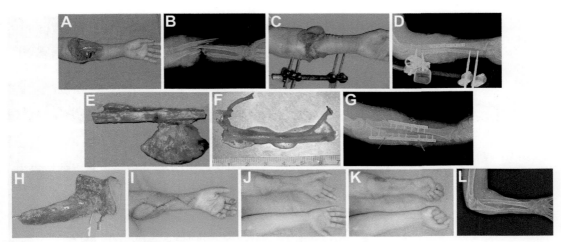

Fig. 4. A 23-year-old man sustained incomplete amputation of the left forearm caused by a punch-out machine. (*A*) The injury involved a significant segmental defect in the proximal forearm with both radial and ulnar arteries crushed, and flexor and extensor muscle groups were ruptured. The superficial radial and ulnar nerves maintained continuity while severely crushed, and the median nerve had a defect. (*B*) The plain radiograph showed a comminuted radius and ulna fracture with significant defects. (*C*) Both ulnar and radial arteries, their venae comitantes, and two subcutaneous veins were repaired. The superficial radial nerve was repaired. The two ends of the median nerve were tagged with nylon sutures at an easily accessible plane for later nerve grafting. Myorrhaphy was done for flexor muscles. (*D*) The radius bone was shortened and fixed with a plate, whereas the ulnar bone was shortened and stabilized with an external fixator filling the bone defect temporarily with bone cement loaded with antibiotics. (*E*) After 3 weeks, simultaneous reconstruction was done with vascularized fibular bone to reconstruct the ulnar bone. (*F*) The median nerve defect was reconstructed using a cable sural nerve graft. (*G*) Immediate postoperative radiograph shows fibular flap (*arrows*). (*H*) Six months later, delayed reconstruction using free functioning gracilis muscle transfer was done to restore thumb and finger flexion. (*I*) Immediate postoperative view. (*J, K*) Four years after injury, the patient can make a fist with pinch and grip strength of approximately 7.3kg and 15.4 kg, respectively. (*L*) Final postoperative radiograph. (*Modified from* Woo SH. Practical tips to improve efficiency and success in upper limb replantation. Plast Reconstr Surg. 2019;144(5):878e-911e, [figure 11].)

This part of the treatment focuses on refining both functional and aesthetic outcomes by addressing any residual deficits. The selection of the most suitable flap for reconstruction also forms a crucial part of this process.

The incidence of delayed reconstruction varies widely ranging from as low as 2.9% to as high as 93.2%[37] and commonly addresses problems related to tendons, bone/joints, soft tissue coverage, nerves, and scar contractures, in descending order of frequency.[38] When examining different levels of amputation, delayed reconstructions include tenolysis for replantations from the distal forearm to the wrist, free functioning muscle transfer (FFMT) for replantations between the elbow and mid-forearm, and soft tissue coverage for upper arm replantations.[38]

Indications

Delayed free flap reconstruction is indicated in a variety of scenarios after replantation. These include using free flaps for additional soft tissue coverage, correcting narrow web spaces, managing scar contracture release, rectifying contour depression, and enhancing movement. Free flaps can also fill bone gaps after managing cases of malunion, nonunion, or osteomyelitis and replace stiff joints following replantation. FFMT can restore function to the elbow, wrist, and fingers in instances where minimal recovery has occurred despite comprehensive interventions and extensive rehabilitation.

Considerations Before Performing Delayed Free Flap Reconstruction

Planning for delayed reconstruction from the onset of treatment is essential. Functional enhancement is possible even when full active motion in the joint is not achieved, as long as full passive motion is preserved. Therefore, a postoperative mobilization protocol should be initiated as early as 72 hours after replantation.[17] Daily exercises with a dynamic crane outrigger splint that features metacarpophalangeal (MCP) joint extension block are recommended, along with the use of a nighttime anticlaw splint. This strategy helps prevent

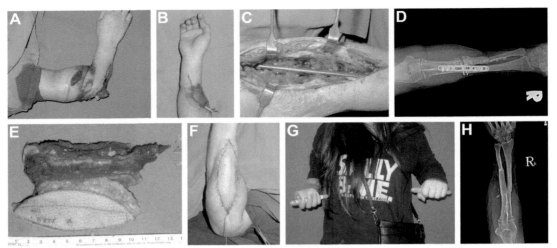

Fig. 5. A 28-year-old woman presented with an incomplete right forearm amputation caused by a hydraulic press machine. (*A*) The patient had a severe crush injury at the mid-forearm with open comminuted fractures of both the radius and ulna. Both radial and ulnar arteries were ruptured, and all muscles in the flexor and extensor groups were torn. (*B*) Following massive debridement, the radial artery was revascularized, and tenodesis was done to the proximal portion of muscles to maintain the finger cascade. Both the radius and the ulna were reduced and internally fixated after bone shortening. (*C, D*) One year after the initial injury, the patient suffered from recurrent episodes of infections involving bone and soft tissue owing to osteomyelitis of the ulnar bone. The infected bone was curetted, and the bone gap was filled with bone cement loaded with antibiotics. (*E, F*) Three months after confirmation of no clinical, radiological, or laboratory signs of infection, the bone cement was removed, and the reconstruction of the ulnar shaft with a free osteocutaneous fibular flap was performed. (*G*) At follow-up 18 months after surgery, the patient demonstrated stable protonation and supination of the forearm without local pain during movement and without evidence of recurrent infection. (*H*) Postoperative radiograph showed a complete bony union of the fibula in the bony gap of the ulna. Courtesy of Ho-Jun Cheon

development of an intrinsic minus deformity, maintain full passive range of motion in the uninjured joints distal to the amputation level, and promote daily use of the replanted digit.[39]

Before proceeding with delayed reconstruction, it is important to ensure soft tissue stability in the previously operated area. Typically, this stability can be achieved within 3 to 6 months following the initial operation, which aligns with the timeline observed in other hand injury patients. Nevertheless, factors, such as infection, delayed wound healing, or graft failure, can prolong this period.

Free Flap Options for Delayed Reconstruction After Replantation

Soft tissue refinement
Soft tissue coverage is one of the earliest interventions in delayed reconstruction, as it is essential before proceeding with any bone, joint, or tendon-based procedures.[5] In cases of replantations at the hand and wrist level, a common challenge is limited thumb movement, which often results in stiffness owing to intrinsic and extrinsic tightness. To achieve an opposable hand, the thumb ray requires an adequate first web space,

basal joint circumduction, and flexible thumb joints. Free flaps, such as radial forearm flaps, ulnar artery flap, lateral arm flap, and first web space of foot flap,[27] can be used for web space coverage after web space release along with arthroplasty or arthrodesis of the thumb basal joint and tenolysis.

Also, free flaps can be used to resurface and provide stable, durable coverage for areas where the wound was initially covered with a skin graft. This helps to promote muscle excursion and offers vascularized soft tissue coverage, which can better manage persistent infections and bone nonunion resulting from high-energy trauma after major limb replantation.

Bone and joint refinement
Reconstruction of radius bone following debridement of osteomyelitis with fibular flap Obtaining bone union is critical for subsequent structural operations, as suboptimal bone healing can lead to malunion, nonunion, or osteomyelitis after replantation.[40] Malunion arises from initial bone misalignment, insufficient immobilization after surgery, repetitive trauma, or bone resorption.[41] Nonunion results from concurrent neurovascular injury, bone deficiency, or infection.[42] Osteomyelitis is

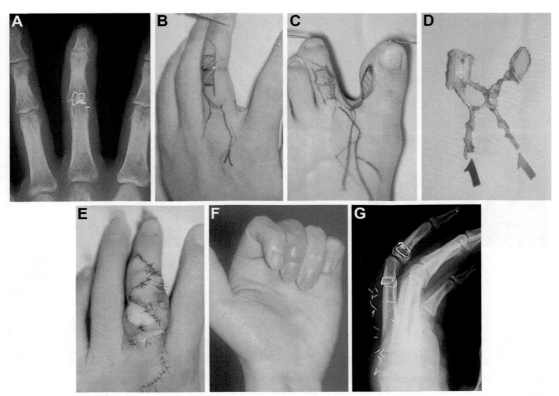

Fig. 6. A 26-year-old man suffered a complete amputation of the left middle finger at the proximal interphalangeal (PIP) joint owing to a power saw injury. The PIP joint was fused during the initial surgery owing to accompanying joint destruction. (*A*) The preoperative radiograph shows the fused PIP joint after the initial replantation. (*B*) Six months after replantation, vascularized toe joint transfer was planned to replace the PIP joint and to provide additional soft tissue coverage on the dorsal aspect of the finger. (*C*) Preoperative design on the ipsilateral foot included a skin flap on the fibular side of the great toe and a PIP joint on the second toe. (*D*) The skin flap and PIP joint were harvested from one pedicle of the first dorsal metatarsal artery and superficial dorsal vein. (*E*) Immediate postoperative photograph. (*F*) Twelve months after the operation, the active range of motion of the PIP joint was 55° with 10° of extension lag. (*G*) Postoperative radiograph.

due to the direct introduction of microorganisms from penetrating trauma or a postoperative soft tissue infection.[43] The first step in the management is to remove any hardware and perform radical debridement of the wound and the bone ends (**Fig. 5**). This may create a gap that may cause unacceptable shortening, requiring the use of a vascularized bone flap. As mentioned in the case, the fibular flap is a good option, but other solutions, such as the medial femoral condyle flap, are increasingly favored owing to their versatility, reliable blood supply, and minimal donor site impact. The medial femoral condyle flap is used for persistent nonunion,[44] significant bone loss in the upper limb, carpal bones, as well as complex bone injuries in the thumb, fingers, and metacarpals.[45]

Reconstruction of proximal interphalangeal joint with vascularized toe joint transfer Joint stiffness

and contractures are another challenge following replantation. Rehabilitation therapy and edema control can often help manage these issues, but in more severe cases, surgical intervention may be necessary. Although stiffness in the distal interphalangeal joints is generally more tolerable owing to their minimal contribution to finger range of motion, contractures in the proximal interphalangeal (PIP) and MCP joints may require procedures like capsulotomy, capsulectomy, arthrodesis, or arthroplasty. Among these, contractures in the PIP joint are most frequently observed after replantation. Vascularized joint transfer from the toe PIP joint has emerged as a promising intervention (**Fig. 6**), particularly suitable for younger patients or those involved in manual labor.[46,47] This technique offers a robust and long-lasting solution, with potential for growth and concurrent reconstruction of composite tissue loss, surpassing traditional methods.

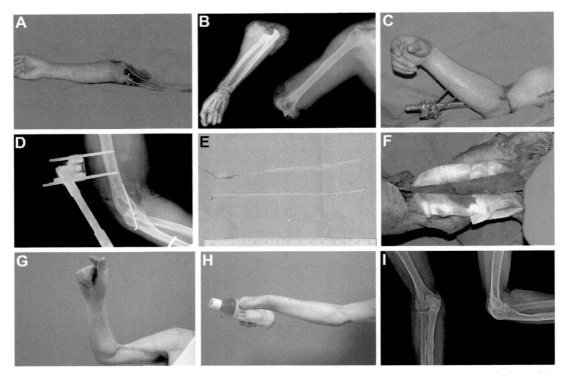

Fig. 7. A 43-year-old man presented with a complete amputation at the elbow level owing to a belt machine injury. (*A*) A traction avulsion injury resulted in all nerves being avulsed from the right upper arm. (*B*) The plain radiograph revealed dislocations of the elbow joint. (*C, D*) Initial operative procedures included radial artery repair, vein graft repair of the ruptured ulnar artery, and extensive debridement of arm and forearm necrotic muscles. The elbow joint with an intact joint surface was temporarily fixated using K-wires and an external fixator to preserve joint function. (*E*) Six months later, sural nerve grafts were used to reconstruct the ulnar and median nerves. (*F*) A free functioning gracilis muscle was transferred to restore elbow flexion. (*G, H*) Fifteen years after the operation, transferred muscle has the power to function against resistance, with 0° to 100° range of motion of the elbow. (*I*) Postoperative radiograph. (Woo SH. Replantation Strategies of the Hand and Upper Extremity. In: Chung KC. Grabb and Smith's Plastic Surgery, 8th Edition. LWW; 2020. p. 839-853.)

Nerve and tendon refinement

Restoring elbow flexion using a free functioning gracilis muscle transfer FFMT is a critical procedure in delayed reconstruction after severe muscle and nerve loss following amputation (**Fig. 7**). FFMT is indicated for patients with complete loss of arm flexors, including biceps and brachialis with disruption of musculocutaneous nerve and complete loss of forearm flexors or extensors with disruption of the innervating nerves without local muscle or tendon available for transfer.[48] For type III avulsion amputation of the forearm or upper arm, it is the only option, as primary nerve repair has minimal benefits for either intrinsic or extrinsic muscle recovery.[22] However, it might not be the optimal choice when a single flexor or extensor compartment is lost, as multiple tendon transfers could offer better results.

The success of FFMT is contingent on injury severity, condition of the innervating nerve,

recipient bed state, and overlying soft tissue coverage. Therefore, FFMT is performed electively, following complete bone and soft tissue healing, usually after a substantial rehabilitation period of more than a year. During the interval, a secondary operation may be carried out to reconstruct the median and ulnar nerves to facilitate sensory recovery and potential intrinsic hand function using a cable nerve graft or vascularized nerve graft.[48]

For FFMT, the gracilis muscle is anatomically optimal and is widely used for its adequate size, shape, reliable vascular pedicle, suitable motor nerve, excellent excursion, and muscle strength. Other options include the rectus femoris muscle or latissimus dorsi muscle. In forearm reconstructions, the anterior interosseous nerve is used for flexor digitorum profundus replacement, and the posterior interosseous nerve is used for extensor digitorum communis replacement. If both the flexor and the extensor of the forearm require reconstruction, the process should start with the extensor, followed by the flexor 4 to 6 months later. Active extension is generally easier to achieve when there is a lack of a strong antagonistic flexor. Conversely, if the flexor side is reconstructed first, it often poses difficulties in attaining adequate finger and wrist extension during rehabilitation.[48,49] For a traumatized and destroyed biceps muscle, the musculocutaneous nerve serves as the donor motor nerve for reconstruction.

Despite the benefits, FFMT after arm replantation has a higher failure rate owing to factors like crushed or contaminated beds and unhealthy donor motor nerves. Furthermore, optimal hand function is not guaranteed because of potential intrinsic muscle paralysis and forearm deformity. Nonetheless, FFMT often results in a functional hand that is more acceptable to patients than amputation or limb prosthesis.

SUMMARY

The restoration of vascularity in replantation marks just the first step on the path to recovery following catastrophic upper extremity injuries. Comprehensive planning is essential for determining the appropriate approach to simultaneous and delayed reconstructions using free flaps. Although free flaps form an integral part of this process, they are not a panacea. Successful reconstruction necessitates preceding and adjunctive procedures along with the free flap. If there are no contraindications, the ultimate aim is to optimize the function of the upper limb replantation, a goal to which free flaps can significantly contribute.

CLINICS CARE POINTS

- Simultaneous free flap reconstruction is a critical tool in replantation surgery. It provides a vascular conduit in cases with vessel defects and offers vascularized coverage for wounds that expose essential structures.
- Arterialized venous flaps can provide essential vessel conduits and soft tissue coverage in digit replantation. By restoring anatomic structures, this technique aids in ensuring the survival of the amputated digit or hand and allows faster wound healing.
- Delayed free flap reconstruction primarily focuses on enhancing function. Incorporating functioning muscle, bone, joint, and nerve components effectively improves the range of motion in the hand and extremity,

provides skeletal stability, and corrects deformities. Soft tissue flaps can address narrow web spaces, manage scar contractures, and rectify contour depressions.

ACKNOWLEDGMENTS

The authors express their profound gratitude to the dedicated staff of the W Institute for Hand and Reconstructive Microsurgery for their tireless commitment to emergency replantation surgery. Special acknowledgment is extended to Dr Ho-Jun Cheon, Dr Youngwoo Kim, Dr Dong-Ho Kang, Dr Hyunjae Nam, Dr Myung-Jae Yoo, Dr Byoung Jin Kim, and Dr Jinhee Choi for their invaluable contributions.

DISCLOSURE

The authors have nothing to disclose.

REFERENCES

1. Lister G, Scheker L. Emergency free flaps to the upper extremity. J Hand Surg Am 1988;13(1):22–8.
2. Derderian CA, Olivier W-AM, Baux G, et al. Microvascular free-tissue transfer for traumatic defects of the upper extremity: a 25-year experience. J Reconstr Microsurg 2003;19(07):455–62.
3. Ninkovic M, Mooney EK, Ninkovic M, et al. A new classification for the standardization of nomenclature in free flap wound closure. Plast Reconstr Surg 1999;103(3):903–14.
4. Yu J-C, Shieh S-J, Lee J-W, et al. Secondary procedures following digital replantation and revascularisation. Br J Plast Surg 2003;56(2):125–8.
5. Sabapathy SR, Bhardwaj P. Secondary procedures in replantation. Semin Plast Surg 2013;27(4): 198–204.
6. Godina M. Early Microsurgical Reconstruction of Complex Trauma of the Extremities. Plast Reconstr Surg 1986;78(3):285–92.
7. Tsai T-M, Matiko JD, Breidenbach W, et al. Venous flaps in digital revascularization and replantation. J Reconstr Microsurg 1987;3(02):113–9.
8. Woo SH, Kim K-C, Lee G-J, et al. A retrospective analysis of 154 arterialized venous flaps for hand reconstruction: an 11-year experience. Plast Reconstr Surg 2007;119(6):1823–38.
9. De SD, Sebastin SJ. Considerations in flap selection for soft tissue defects of the hand. Clin Plast Surg 2019;46(3):393–406.
10. Sabapathy SR, Bajantri B. Indications, selection, and use of distant pedicled flap for upper limb reconstruction. Hand Clin 2014;30(2):185–99.
11. Hsu C-C, Lin Y-T, Lin C-H, et al. Immediate emergency free anterolateral thigh flap transfer for the

mutilated upper extremity. Plast Reconstr Surg 2009; 123(6):1739–47.

12. Sundine M, Scheker L. A comparison of immediate and staged reconstruction of the dorsum of the hand. J Hand Surg Am 1996;21(2):216–21.

13. Byrd HS, Spicer TE, Cierney G III. Management of open tibial fractures. Plast Reconstr Surg 1985; 76(5):719–28.

14. Harrison BL, Lakhiani C, Lee MR, et al. Timing of traumatic upper extremity free flap reconstruction: a systematic review and progress report. Plast Reconstr Surg 2013;132(3):591–6.

15. Kolker AR, Kasabian AK, Karp NS, et al. Fate of free flap microanastomosis distal to the zone of injury in lower extremity trauma. Plast Reconstr Surg 1997; 99(4):1068–73.

16. Bendon CL, Giele HP. Success of free flap anastomoses performed within the zone of trauma in acute lower limb reconstruction. J Plast Reconstr Aesthet Surg 2016;69(7):888–93.

17. Woo SH. Replantation Strategies of the Hand and Upper Extremity. In: Chung KC, editor. Grabb and Smith's plastic surgery. 8th edition. Philadelphia, PA: Lippincott Williams & Wilkins; 2019. p. 839–53.

18. Brandt K, Khouri RK, Upton J. Free flaps as flow-through vascular conduits for simultaneous coverage and revascularization of the hand or digit. Plast Reconstr Surg 1996;98(2):321–7.

19. Woo SH, Jeong J, Seul J. Resurfacing relatively large skin defects of the hand using arterialized venous flaps. J Hand Surg Am 1996;21(2):222–9.

20. Woo SH, Lee YK, Kim JY, et al. Palmaris longus tendocutaneous arterialized venous free flap to reconstruct the interphalangeal collateral ligament in composite defects. J Hand Surg Eur 2018;43(5):518–23.

21. Lee Y-K, Kim J-Y, Sagong S-Y, et al. Functional Reconstruction of the Digit using Palmaris Longus Tendocutaneous Arterialized Venous Free Flap. J Korean Soc Surg Hand 2014;19(3):136–44.

22. Chuang D, Lai J-B, Cheng S-L, et al. Traction avulsion amputation of the major upper limb: a proposed new classification, guidelines for acute management, and strategies for secondary reconstruction. Plast Reconstr Surg 2001;108(6):1624–38.

23. Lee C-H, Han S-K, Dhong E-S, et al. The fate of microanastomosed digital arteries after successful replantation. Plast Reconstr Surg 2005;116(3):805–10.

24. Yang J-W, Kim J-S, Lee D-C, et al. The radial artery superficial palmar branch flap: a modified free thenar flap with constant innervation. J Reconstr Microsurg 2010;26(08):529–38.

25. Lee Y, Woo SH, Kim YW, et al. Free Flaps for Soft Tissue Reconstruction of Digits. Hand Clin 2020 Feb; 36(1):85–96.

26. Tsai T-M, Sabapathy SR, Martin D. Revascularization of a finger with a thenar mini-free flap. J Hand Surg Am 1991;16(4):604–6.

27. Kim KS, Kim ES, Hwang JH, et al. Fingertip reconstruction using the hypothenar perforator free flap. J Plast Reconstr Aesthet Surg 2013 Sep;66(9): 1263–70.

28. Takami H, Takahashi S, Ando M. Use of the dorsalis pedis free flap for reconstruction of the hand. Hand 1983;2:173–8.

29. Narushima M, Iida T, Kaji N, et al. Superficial circumflex iliac artery pure skin perforator-based superthin flap for hand and finger reconstruction. J Plast Reconstr Aesthet Surg 2016 Jun;69(6):827–34.

30. Woo SH, Choi B-C, Oh S-J, et al. Classification of the first web space free flap of the foot and its applications in reconstruction of the hand. Plast Reconstr Surg 1999;103(2):508–17.

31. Woo SH. Practical tips to improve efficiency and success in upper limb replantation. Plast Reconstr Surg 2019;144(5):878e–911e.

32. Kimata Y, Uchiyama K, Ebihara S, et al. Anterolateral thigh flap donor-site complications and morbidity. Plast Reconstr Surg 2000;106(3):584–9.

33. Chang N-J, Waughlock N, Kao D, et al. Efficient design of split anterolateral thigh flap in extremity reconstruction. Plast Reconstr Surg 2011;128(6): 1242–9.

34. Yousif JN, Ye Z, Grunert BK, et al. Analysis of the distribution of cutaneous perforators in cutaneous flaps. Plast Reconstr Surg 1998;101(1):72–84.

35. Wei F-C, Chen H-C, Chuang C-C, et al. Fibular osteoseptocutaneous flap: anatomic study and clinical application. Plast Reconstr Surg 1986;78(2): 191–9.

36. Sauerbier M, Unglaub F. Perforator flaps in the upper extremity. Clin Plast Surg 2010;37(4):667–76.

37. Wang H. Secondary surgery after digit replantation: its incidence and sequence. Microsurgery 2002 2002;22(2):57–61.

38. Fufa D, Lin CH, Lin YT, et al. Secondary reconstructive surgery following major upper extremity replantation. Plast Reconstr Surg 2014;134(4):713–20.

39. Scheker LR, Chesher SP, Netscher DT, et al. Functional results of dynamic splinting after transmetacarpal, wrist, and distal forearm replantation. J Hand Surg Br 1995;20(5):584–90.

40. Whitney TM, Lineaweaver WC, Buncke HJ, et al. Clinical results of bony fixation methods in digital replantation. J Hand Surg Am 1990;15(2):328–34.

41. Chiou GJ, Chang J. Refinements and secondary surgery after flap reconstruction of the traumatized hand. Hand Clin 2014;30(2):211–23.

42. Ring D. Malunion and nonunion of the metacarpals and phalanges. Instr Course Lect 2006;55:121–8.

43. Honda H, McDonald JR. Current recommendations in the management of osteomyelitis of the hand and wrist. J Hand Surg Am 2009;34(6):1135–6.

44. Del Piñal F, García-Bernal FJ, Regalado J, et al. Vascularised corticoperiosteal grafts from the medial

femoral condyle for difficult non-unions of the upper limb. J Hand Surg Eur 2007;32(2):135–42.

45. Hsu C-C, Tseng J, Lin Y-T. Chimeric Medial Femoral Condyle Osteocutaneous Flap for Reconstruction of Multiple Metacarpal Defects. J Hand Surg Am 2018; 43(8):781.e1–9.

46. Chen HY, Lin YT, Lo S, et al. Vascularised toe proximal interphalangeal joint transfer in posttraumatic finger joint reconstruction: the effect of skin paddle design on extensor lag. J Plast Reconstr Aesthet Surg 2014;67(1):56–62.

47. Woo SH, Seul J, Kim JS. Vascularized toe joint transfers for hand reconstruction. J Korean Soc Reconstr Hand Surg 1999;4(1):73–81.

48. Lin SH, Chuang DC, Hattori Y, et al. Traumatic major muscle loss in the upper extremity: reconstruction using functioning free muscle transplantation. J Reconstr Microsurg 2004;20(3):227–35.

49. Chuang DC, Strauch RJ, Wei FC. Technical considerations in two-stage functioning free muscle transplantation reconstruction of both flexor and extensor functions of the forearm. Microsurgery 1994;15(5):338–43.

9780443130137